Legal & Disclaimer

changes are periodically made to this book as and when needed. Where appropriate and/or necessary, you must consult a professional (including but not limited to your doctor, attorney, financial advisor or such other professional advisor) before using any of the suggested remedies, techniques, or information in this book.

Upon using the contents and information contained in this book, you agree to hold harmless the Author from and against any damages, costs, and expenses, including any legal fees potentially resulting from the application of any of the information provided by this book. This disclaimer applies to any loss, damages or injury caused by the use and application, whether directly or indirectly, of any advice or information presented, whether for breach of contract, tort, negligence, personal injury, criminal intent, or under any other cause of action.

You agree to accept all risks of using the information presented inside this book.

You agree that by continuing to read this book, where appropriate and/or necessary, you shall consult a professional (including but not limited to your doctor, attorney, or financial advisor or such other advisor as needed) before using any of the suggested remedies, techniques, or information in this book.

Table of Contents

Chapter 6: Soups and Stews Recipes 106

Introduction

Greetings! It's great that you have finally found time to join us here!

As you know, nowadays a lot of people in our world spend majority of their life on the go. Most of us are overwhelmed with work not only during the week, but on the weekends, as well. This makes us depend on things like fast food. You want to eat healthy, but you just can't afford to spend countless hours cooking? Well, then the Crock Pot might just be the perfect option for you! It saves you a great deal of time, thus helping you to stay on schedule and minimizing the time you spend cooking. Being the owner of the Crock Pot is one thing, but knowing how to maximize the health benefits of using it is another! If you have decided to stick to the Ketogenic diet chances are you have already encountered many challenges. But what if I tell you that the Crock Pot that is standing on the counter in your kitchen is a magic wand you have simply forgotten about? Are you looking for recipe ideas that would be delicious and also follow the rules of the ketogenic diet? In this case, I assure you, my friend, you have found just the right book!

This book is perfect for food-loving Crock Pot owners that follow the ketogenic diet, as it provides a lot of useful information regarding the state-of-the-art capabilities of the Crock Pot and the benefits of the ketogenic diet. The ketogenic diet does include lots of «complicated» rules, but it will be much easier to follow them using this book and the recipes in it. The recipes of the Keto Crock Pot Cook Book are rather simple, accessible, adaptable and easy to understand and to make in the Crock Pot that is already in your kitchen! Now it will be so much easier to enjoy your favorite foods! The recipes in the cookbook are divided into chapters, so that finding them becomes a piece of cake. So, let's cook together and have some fun!

Chapter 1: the Keto Diet & the Crock Pot

What Is the Ketogenic Diet?

A ketogenic or simply a keto diet is a popular modern low-carb diet. It forces the body to use small fuel molecules that are called "ketones" as the main energy source. The liver breaks down fats into fatty acids and ketones, when the blood sugar levels are low. The glucose is actually the easiest molecule in the body to break down and that is why it is usually used as the main energy source. If a person eats food high in carbs, the organism begins to produce both insulin and, of course, glucose. Insulin is generated by the body to bring the glucose into the bloodstream taking it around your body. There is no need for the body to process the fats since the glucose supplies energy. In this case, fats are stored in the body. Lowering the consumption of carbohydrates induces ketosis in the body. The ketones are generated by the body if a person consumes a small amount of carbs that are quickly broken down and a plenty of protein. The ketones produced by the liver are used to fuel important organs, including the brain. The latter needs a lot of fuel to fulfill even the simplest daily functions, but cannot run on fats, only on ketones or glucose. The main aim of a ketogenic diet is to force the body into the metabolic state. The human's body is incredibly adaptable to everything an individual puts into it – as soon as a person overloads the body with fat, taking away all carbohydrates, it quickly begins to process and burn the ketones. The optimal keto level is a great way to stay healthy and lose excess weight, as it has both mental and physical benefits. This book can be your assistant on the journey to the keto-diet world.

What You Can Eat during the Ketogenic Diet

If you are an individual that is not completely sure what is allowed during a keto diet and what must be strictly avoided, this part of our book will be of tremendous help for you! Sticking to any diet isn't easy, I think most women know what I'm talking about. It gets more complicated when you have no idea what you should consume during the day. It may become a real challenge to keep a keto diet if it is new for you. But the recipes, meal plans and shopping lists included in this book will make your keto-life so much easier. Remember the main rule - following this diet you have to be focused on eating real food that is also low in carbs. A short list of allowed products and of those, you must avoid provided below. An easy visual guide of products that fit in with the requirements of a ketogenic diet is amazing for beginners who would like to make the right decisions on what exactly to eat and, of course, shop for.

-   ***Oils and fats***

Fats must make up the majority of the calories you consume in a day. Here you have the options to choose from, what you prefer and what you don't like. Basic lovely dressings, sauces and toppings could be added to chicken or beef in any combination your heart desires! Fats are significant for the organism, but too many of them could potentially have adverse effects on your body. The ketogenic diets involves the consumption of the following types of fats: saturated (like ghee, butter, green bacon, coconut oil); as well as monounsaturated fats (nut, avocado, olive oil). Be careful with polyunsaturated fats (eat fatty fish and animal protein, but strictly avoid margarine spreads). Trans-fats – try to avoid entirely! This fat has an altered chemical composition and can lead to heart disease. Keep a balance between the levels of omega 6's and omega 3's, consuming lots of tuna, wild salmon, trout will help you to keep the balance necessary for your health. Be careful with the consumption of seeds and nuts as they are a source of omega 3's. Almonds, pine nuts, walnuts, corn oil fall into this category. The food that could be ideal for your keto diet is – animal fat, fatty fish, lard, avocado, ghee, butter, mayo, macadamia/avocado/olive/coconut oil, cocoa and coconut butter, vitellus, tallow. That list also includes grass-fed meat, such as lamb and beef, seafood and wild-caught fish, pastured pork, and some of the animal organs, namely heart, liver or kidneys.

- ***Protein***

Chose the dark meat because it contains more fat than the white meat. If you prefer to eat red meat there is not so much to elude here, eat a ribeye or some ground beef. In terms of sausages you have to avoid buying those with added sugar. You shouldn't consume too much protein either, because it can cause the levels of ketone production to decrease, which means your body will have to rely on glucose. Here are some examples of protein you are allowed to consume: fish (flounder, cod, mackerel, halibut etc.); shellfish (lobster, mussels, clams, oysters); beef (steak, stew meat, roasts etc.); eggs; pork, liver, kidney, heart etc.; poultry; goat; lamb; turkey; sausages and bacon (read the labels); nut butter (unsweetened and natural nuts, try to find the versions that are higher in fats).

- *Fruit and veggies*

The best vegetables for this diet are green and leafy, as they are grown above the ground. When it comes to veggies that grow below the ground, consume them in moderation. Actually, if there is a vegetable you really love or crave, the rule here is to just consume it in moderation. The vegetables that you are allowed to eat are: spinach, lettuce, chives, radicchio, endive, etc.; radishes, kale, kale turnip, asparagus, summer squash, cucumber, bamboo shoots. When eating berries try to control the levels of carbs in them.

- *Dairy (milk)products*

Milk products are usually consumed by an individual within a keto diet in a combination with a variety of other variety of products. The most part of foods consumed by an individual must be based on veggies and added fats. Favored are organic, raw products, high in fats. For those individuals who are lactose sensitive, it is important to try and consume pasteurized and hard dairy. The allowed dairy products are: mozzarella, blue, brie, Monterey Jack, Greek yogurt, spreadable, hard cheese (Swiss or etc.), mayo, mascarpone, sour crème etc.

- ***Seeds and nuts***

You may consume seeds and nuts, especially when they are parched, using them as appetizers or as flavorings to the main dish. If possible try to exclude peanuts, as these nuts are legumes. I think, you know, the nuts are a perfect source of fat, that's why when consuming them you must carefully balance the levels of protein you consume. Next time around, you open a pack of nuts, remember what you are allowed to eat: Brazil and macadamia nuts, pecans, almonds, walnuts, pine nuts, peanuts and hazelnuts.

- ***Spices and cooking***

Sauces and seasoning are an intricate part of the keto diet, but the good news is that you can continue to make/use your favorites. There is no reason to list all of the allowed spices, as there is a great number of them. Some of them are amazing to use, however the others – have a high glycemic index. The sea salt is preferable over table salt. The spices that are allowed during this type of a diet are: cinnamon, chili powder, cayenne pepper, Greek oregano, cumin, cilantro, basil, rosemary, parsley, thyme. Be sure, you can consume pepper and salt without worrying.

- *Sauces and condiments*

The sauces as well as other condiments are at the twilight zone on keto diet. This is due to the fact that if you try to strictly stick to the keto diet, the premade sauces must be avoided altogether, because they may contain the commonly obtained sugars and sweeteners that aren't appropriable on the diet. The sauces or some gravies that you select to cook must be based on xanthan gum or guar. They are much lower in carbs than the others. Also, if you are buying a premade sauce, read the label attentively! The allowed sauces are: mustard, Dijon mustard, ketchup, hot sauce, mayo, sauerkraut (without sugar or low in sugar), relish, Worcestershire Sauce, salad dressings (the fattier ones), flavored syrups (with permitted sweeteners).

- *Sweeteners*

It will be not so easy to keep this keto diet for those individuals who love sweets. But doing this is possible and you do have two options – either keeping your sweets intake on almost a zero level or using the substitutes. If you still wish to consume sweeteners, chose the fluid versions. You may also identify which one tastes better for you as there is a great number of diverse sorts and new altered substitutions of them. The most popular are: Stevia (preferred in liquid form), sucralose (rather sweet substitution), monk fruit, erythritol etc.

- ***Beverages***

Among the preferred beverages when sticking to a keto diet are: coffee with coconut milk or cream, water, black or herbal tea.

What you can't eat during the ketogenic diet

And now, when you already have a clear idea about which products you might consume during a ketogenic diet, it is the time to complete the list of forbidden products. If you still are not sure about the products that aren't keto appropriate, this list of limitations will definitely help you:

-    Sugar – it can be found almost in all soda, mostly all juice, the plurality of sports drinks, sweet candies (even if these are your favorite ones!), chocolate, ice cream.
-    Grains - the wheat products (these include also bread and buns), gruels, pasta, cakes, paddy and corn, beer must be avoided too. This also includes the whole grains like rye, wheat, buckwheat, barleycorn and quinoa.
-    Starch – during the keto diet an individual has to avoid some vegetables (like potatoes, yams) oats, etc.

Only some of the vegetables are edible but in moderation.

- Trans-fats – paste-like butter substitutes, like margarine and other variations of it should be avoided as they contain hydrogenated fats. These are also bad for our health.

- Fruit – a person who is sticking to the low-starch diet must avoid consuming large fruits like apples, bananas, oranges, because they are extremely high in sugar. Consume the berries in moderation, check the labels if you buy them at the store.

- Low-fat foods – these products are usually much higher in carbs and sugar than the other full-fat versions. Be sure you read the package at the store to avoid making mistakes.

- Factory-farmed pork and fish - are high in inflammatory omega 6 fatty acids, farmed fish could include PCBs, and you must avoid fish high in mercury.

- Milk isn't recommended for a number of reasons. First of all, it is rather complication to digest; it lacks the "good" bacteria and even contains hormones. Also it is high in starch (containing about 5 grams of starch per 100 ml). As for coffee and tea, if you prefer to drink them with milk, substitute milk with cream, but, like with everything else, in moderate amounts.

- Sweet and alcoholic drinks (sweet wine, beer, all the mixed drinks, etc.).

- Pistachios and cashews - consume rarely as they're very high in starch (for example, two handfuls of cashews contains a daily maximum for starch intake).

Benefits of the ketogenic diet

There is a huge variety of diets that come and go, but the ketogenic or the keto diet having been developed not so long ago is gaining increasing popularity. This type of diet is fully based on your knowing the theory and understanding nutritional science and human physiology. When in most diets an individual relies upon counting the consumed calories, sorting the portions, avoiding fats strictly, the keto diet works in a completely different manner, by changing the «fuel source» that an individual uses to obtain energy and be fit all day long 7/24. But the ketogenic diet wasn't greeted by all scientists with open arms right away. Since 2002 more than 15 studies were conducted based on the rules and principals of the ketogenic diet. Almost everyone has proved that this diet was at the top three of all diets. Next, I will list the advantages of a keto diet, they are 1 – the ketogenic diet kills the appetite: hunger was always the adverse reaction to any diet you have already practiced. This is the main reason why individuals dislike and terminate the diets. Consuming fats and low-carb products reduces the appetite. 2 – Sticking to the keto diet allows you to lose more weight than with other diets: the main reason being that the low-carbs tend to get rid of the excessive liquid stored in the human body. People, who stick to this keto diet can lose weight twice as fast. The keto-diets seem to be effective for up to 5 months, after this time an individual's body begins to push back, it occurs usually when people give up and begin to eat the old way. 3 – Getting rid of the fat in the abdominal area. The bodies of the individuals differ from each other. People have two main fat storage locations – in the abdomen, the visceral fat, and, the subcutaneous fat, stored under the skin. The keto diet reduces the visceral fat of the organism, the increased amounts of which could lead to insulin stamina, distraction, and are the mainspring of metabolic indigestion. 4 – The levels of fat moieties called triglycerides tend to go down to zero. 5 – The level of the high-density lipoprotein (HDL) that is also called the «good» cholesterol could be increased due to the keto diet. The higher is the level of the individual's HDL, the lower is the risk of suffering from heart disease. Eating fat is the best way to increase your HDL level. 6 – The ketogenic diet reduces the insulin levels and the level of blood sugar because an individual avoids consuming the carbs that are dragged down into glucose in the gastrointestinal tract. 7 – The ketogenic diet reduces the high blood pressure and as a result, the risk of saccharine disease gets lower. 8 – It is a good way to fight against the metabolic syndrome. The last one is the medical condition that is also combined with heart problems risk and diabetes. 9 – The keto diet is good for brain disorders because of the therapeutic effect. A part of an individual's brain can incinerate the glucose only. But the others one can also burn ketones that are mostly formed, for example during starvation. The method of the keto diet was applied earlier for treating epilepsy in kids. Nowadays this diet is being used for treating Parkinson's and Alzheimer's disease.

Keto for beginners

Now you know a lot about the ketogenic diet, what to eat and what products are not allowed. I hope you have already understood how healthy this type of diet is and you are going to stick to it, just like I will. Sure, every beginning is rather complicated, but if you have a Crock Pot in the kitchen it solves the majority of problems that could arise. In order to decrease the difficultness of the keto beginning, try to consume keto foods slowly, week after week. Remember that the keto diet could change the mineral and water balance in the body, that's why you may add some extra salt to the consumed foods. It is essential to eat until you feel fool, avoiding restricting calories too much. A short list of frequently asked questions about the keto diet using the Crock Pot will definitely help you at the starting stage:

- Is it dangerous for health to stop eating carbs completely? – No, after some months (2-3) you might eat them occasionally, but then return to the keto diet cooking your meals in the Crock Pot.
- I have heard ketosis is dangerous. Is it true? – Don't mix up the ketoacidos with ketosis. Ketoacidosis occurs in uncontrolled diabetes. By the way, using your Crock Pot for cooking is already much healthier than usual cooking.
- Do I have to count my calories? – Be attentive of them, read the labels at the markets and avoid trans-fats and sweeteners.
- Can I prepare the dishes late in the evening to eat them in the morning for breakfast? – Sure,

cook in your great helper (the Crock Pot) and then turn on WARM, in the morning you will have the warm breakfast at the table.

- How much protein should I eat? – Don't eat too much, the high levels of it could increase the insulin level in the body. Consume not more than 30-40% of general calorie intake.
- Is it possible to combine the keto diet with the fast pace of my life as I work all day long 7/24? – Sure! This keto Crock Pot cookbook is definitely for you! Save time, eat well and stick to the diet!

Moreover, the keto diet using the crock pot is great for diabetics, people who are overweight, busy men and women, moms and dads.

Crock Pot. What is it?

I feel like everyone has heard of a Crock Pot at least once in their life. It appeared in 1970 and was marketed as a bean cooker. But as it was modified people started to use it to heat up food and keep it warm for prolonged periods of time. And look how far we've come; people are cooking delicious healthy meals in it. It is a perfect small kitchen appliance that consists of a glass lid, a porcelain or a ceramic pot (it is inside of the heating unit) and, of course, a heating element. The modern Crock Pots could be of an oval or a round shape and of various sizes, from small to large. All the Crock Pots have two settingss: LOW (it corresponds to the temperature of 200°F mostly) and HIGH (up to the temperature of 300°F). The WARMing option that is among the options of the majority of the Crock Pots nowadays allows to keep the prepared dishes warm for a long periods of time. Some of the Crock Pot models have a timer that allows you to control cooking time if you are busy.

What Are the Benefits of Using the Crock Pot?

What is the most difficult thing for you in the kitchen? You spend too much time in the kitchen when you might go to the cinema with friends? You spend too much money for products and your ideas for what to prepare today are running out? I know the solution to all your problems… It is the Crock Pot!

Firstly, it is possible to prepare meals when you are not at home. During those hectic family mornings, just throw all the ingredients together following the recipe, switch the machine on and go work.

Secondly, you don't like washing the dishes? Neither do I! Just clean the Crock Pot and the plates after delicious meals. That's all! Using the Crock Pot means having fewer dishes to wash.

Thirdly, the Crock Pot cooks the delicious meals and saves your money!

These meals taste even better than usual and also you can keep the leftovers in the refrigerator to eat later.

How perfect are the spice flavors if you eat the dishes right after cooking! You might taste the cayenne pepper, cumin, ginger and other favorite spices of yours. Buy simple products and follow the cookbook. It is easy!

Fourth benefit, the Crock Pot is the best way to keep your meal tender and always warm.

Fifth, the Crock Pot reduces calories and fat. No oil (just olive or avocado oil), no frying is necessary.

Six, step by step preparation.

Step by step preparation facilitates the everyday cooking especially for those who are not great fans of this process. In most recipes, all the ingredients are added at one time to the Crock Pot.

Seven, it is energy saving. It requires less electricity than the usual oven.

The flexibility of the Crock Pot is benefit number eight. You can take it on a trip, put it on the kitchen table or somewhere else. It doesn't need that much space.

And finally, benefit number nine is in the large quantities of prepared meals. Most of these recipes make large quantities of the end products, so you may feed an entire family and even freeze for tomorrow to make easy and quick lunches or suppers.

So, are you already looking for some recipes to get started? Check my great keto Crock Pot cookbook and you'll find the best and most delicious dishes here! Cooking keto recipes in the Crock Pot will help you to fit cooking into your daily schedule and stay healthy. After a long working day, you'll be back home and a delicious meal will be there waiting for you.

Chapter 2: Breakfast Recipes

Keto Crock Pot Turkey Stuffed Peppers

The delectable keto Crock Pot turkey stuffed peppers is a great healthy recipe, matching for family breakfast on weekend, as well as during the day. If you have too little time to cook it right now in the Crock Pot, you can freeze the peppers and prepare them in the Crock Pot later. Instead of ground turkey, you may use the ground beef if you wish.

Ingredients (7 servings):

olive oil	1 tablespoon
ground turkey	1 lb
onion	1 pcs
garlic	1 clove
green bell peppers	4 pcs
tomato sauce/pasta sauce (low carb)	24 oz jar

water   1/2 cup

Directions:

1. Peel and cut the small onion, peel the garlic and press or mince it.
2. Wash the bell peppers, cut off the tops and clean them accurately.
3. Take a medium bowl, put there ground turkey, cut onion, pressed or minced garlic and add pasta sauce.
4. Separate the compound into four equal parts, place the compounds into the prepared cleaned peppers.
5. Spread the olive oil over the Crock Pot bottom and sides put the peppers to the Crock Pot and top them with sauce.
6. Add a little water into the Crock Pot too, cover and cook on LOW for 6-7 hours.
7. Serve with remaining sauce and enjoy!
8. Bon Appetite!

Crock-Pot Keto Artichoke, Spinach

An easy keto recipe with artichoke hearts and frozen spinach is light and hearty. It updates your usual boring morning breakfast with balmy relish. You may serve it with vegetables or keto bread.

Ingredients (6 servings):

jarred artichoke hearts   14 - 15 ounces

spinach (frozen)	10 ounces
cream cheese	8 ounces
Parmesan cheese	1 cup
Garlic	3 cloves

Sea salt and pepper at will

Directions:
1. Peel the garlic, mince it.
2. Grate the cheese.
3. Prepare the frozen spinach, don't defrost them.
4. Drain half of the liquid from the jarred artichokes.
5. Conjoin all the components – artichoke, spinach, cream cheese, Parmesan, minced garlic in the Crock Pot. Savour sea salt and pepper at will.
6. Cap and cook on LOW for two hours. The cheese must be melted.
7. Stir from time to time.
8. Serve with keto bread or vegetables.

Keto Jalapeño Popper

If you prefer jalapeño poppers, a combination of hot peppers with cheese, you are going the right way! I'm sure you'll love this hot recipe that is great for a lot number of family members. If you have a big family, prepare this tasty one with the same ingredients but double the portions and cook this recipe in a large Crock Pot if you have. Serve with your favorite veggies!

Ingredients (7 servings):

cream cheese	16 ounces
mayonnaise	1 cup
green chilies	4 ounces canned
jalapeño chilies	4 ounces canned
Mexican cheese	1/2 cup
mozzarella cheese	1/2 cup
Parmesan cheese	1/4 cup

Directions:
1. Prepare the cream cheese softened and cubed.
2. Drain the green chilies and chop them carefully.
3. Drain the jalapeno chilies and slice them also.
4. Blend the Mexican cheese.
5. Rub the Parmesan and cut mozzarella into cubes.
6. Combine all the ingredients in the bowl, add mayonnaise and stir it thoroughly.
7. Put the mixture into the Crock Pot, cover and cook on LOW 1 hour.
8. Stir the mixture 2-3 times during an hour.
9. Serve warm.
10. Bon Appetite!

Keto Asiago Spinach Dip

Keto asiago spinach dip is a great mixture of simple 5 ingredients for cooking in the Crock Pot! If you haven't tried the asiago cheese yet, it would be perfect finding for you. So easy and full of flavor.

Ingredients (5 servings):

neufchâtel cheese or cream cheese	1 pound
asiago cheese	1 pound
fresh baby spinach	6 ounces
garlic powder	1 teaspoon
Italian seasoning	1/2 teaspoon

Seal salt and pepper to taste

Directions:

1. Shred the asiago cheese, chop the washed fresh baby spinach leaves roughly.
2. Combine in the large bowl the asiago cheese, Neufchâtel cheese, garlic powder, spinach with Italian seasoning and stir carefully.
3. Smooth this to the Crock-Pot, cover and cook on LOW for 2 hours.
4. The spinach must wilt and the asiago cheese must be melted.
5. Stir every 15-20 minutes, to be sure your dish doesn't burn or stick.
6. After 2 hours set the Crock Pot on WARM and serve it!
7. Bon Appetite!

Crock-Pot All in Hot Dip

This recipe needs to use the previously cooked ground beef as well as sausages that could be made previously in the same Crock Pot. Recipes made with American cheese taste especially great! Balmy dip must be served warm! Enjoy great melted cheese in a combination of ground pork and cream celery soup.

Ingredients (6 servings):

Cooked ground beef	1 pound
Cooked sausages	1 pound
cream of chicken soup canned	10.75 ounces
cream of celery soup canned	10.75 ounces
jarred salsa	24 ounces
American cheese	1 pound

Salt and pepper at will

Directions:

1. Shred the American cheese, prepare at hand all the ingredients.
2. Mix in the Crock Pot the ground beef, sausages, cream of chicken soup, cream of celery, shredded American cheese, jarred salsa, salt and pepper at will.
3. Cover and cook everything on HIGH for 2 hours. Stir from time to time.

4. Turn the Crock Pot on WARM to keep it warm and tasty while serving.
5. Bon Appetite!

Keto Venison Tenderloin

If you are from a hunting family or just a fan of venison, don't hesitate to prepare keto venison in the Crock Pot for breakfast! The flavor of venison doesn't leave you indifferent. But you may also prepare this dish of beef tenderloin. Use the dressing mix or do-it-yourself. My mouth has already started to water…

Ingredients (5 servings):

venison tenderloin	2 pounds
cheese cream	10.5 ounces can
cream of chicken soup	10.5 ounces can
ranch dressing mix	1 packet
salt and pepper to taste	

Directions:
1. Slice the venison into 1 inch thick slices.
2. Open the can of cheese cream conjoin it with chicken soup cream, add dressing, salt, and pepper at will, sliced venison at the Crock Pot.
3. Cover and cook on LOW for 5 – 6 hours so the venison must be tender.
4. Stir from time to time during the cooking process.

5. Serve warm.
6. Bon Appetite!

Keto Awesome Pot Roast

I like easy and simple recipes but essential ones. They don't need a plenty of ingredients, are tasty and for all the family members. Here is the simple pork roast recipe for morning breakfast for those who work hard during a day! Don't forget about the keto diet rules.

Ingredients (3 servings):

pork roast such as Boston butt roast   4 pounds

Worcestershire sauce   1/4 cup

seasoned salt   1 teaspoon

Directions:
1. Add a half of the Worcestershire sauce to the Crock pot's bottom.
2. Put the pork in the bottom inside.
3. Spread the remaining sauce over the top of the pork roast.
4. Cover and cook on LOW for 8-10 hours.
5. Take off the pork roast, place it on the plate and shred on slices.
6. Bon Appetite!

Keto Creamy Italian Pork Chops

Keto creamy Italian pork is one of the easiest recipes to prepare for the breakfast. Simple contents and the tasty dish is on the table. You may put the pork into the Crock Pot late in the evening and serve it warm early in the morning. The Italian mix gives a great taste, the other ingredients keep the pork chops tender and moist.

Ingredients (5 servings):

pork chops	6 whole pcs
Dressing (Italian one)	1 package
yellow onion	1 pcs
cream of chicken soup	10.75 ounces can
ground paprika	2 dashes
salt and pepper at will	

Directions:
1. Peel and chop the onion.
2. Spray the bottom and walls of Crock Pot with a little bit of cooking spray.
3. Put down the pork in the Crock Pot, covering it with chopped onions.
4. Take a medium bowl and conjoin there all volume of the envelope of Italian dressing, cream of chicken soup, add salt and pepper, ground paprika.
5. Add the contents over the combination of chopped onions and pork chops in the Crock

Pot, supplement a little bit paprika pinches over the top.

6. Cap and cook on LOW for 4-5 hours.
7. Bon Appetite!

Keto Simple Corned Beef

I decided to cook for the morning the simple corned beef, I took the package with sugar-free ingredients. Be attentive, the corned beef is rather a salty one, if you want to eat less salt, rinse the beef with water. If you have a smaller package of corned beef (ex. 1 pound) than the mentioned dosage, divide the ingredients in a half and cook.

Ingredients (8 servings):

yellow onion	1 large pcs
corned beef (without sugar)	2-pounds
laurel leaf	1 leaf
garlic	3 - 4 whole cloves
water	3/4 cup
Stevia	2 tablespoons
prepared yellow mustard	2 teaspoons
freshly ground black pepper	1/4 teaspoon
salt and pepper at taste	

Directions:
1. Peel and slice the onion. Peel the garlic and mince it.
2. Spray the Crock Pot with cooking spray.
3. Put the sliced onion. Take off the corned beef from the package and wash properly with warm water.
4. Add the beef to the onion pillow. Place the laurel leaf.
5. Take a medium bowl mix there Stevia, water, mustard, salt, pepper and stir together.
6. Pour the mixture over the dish, don't take off the laurel leaf.
7. Cover and cook on HIGH for 5-6 hours.
8. Take off the dish to the place and enjoy!
9. Bon Appetite!

Greek Eggs Breakfast Casserole

I'd like to present you here an amazing mixture of vegetables, Feta cheese, and eggs! Try to taste the Greek eggs breakfast casserole and I'm sure it will be among your favorites forever!

Ingredients (9 servings):

eggs (whisked)	12 pcs
milk	½ cup

salt	½ teaspoon
black pepper	1 teaspoon
Red Onion	1 tablespoon
Garlic	1 teaspoon
Sun-dried tomatoes	½ cup
spinach	2 cups
Feta Cheese	½ cup
pepper at will	

Directions:

1. Peel the onion and garlic and cut them (you may also press the garlic). Cut the spinach. Crush Feta cheese in a little plate.
2. Take a bowl, crack the eggs and whisk them thoroughly.
3. Add to the mixture milk, pepper, salt and stir to combine.
4. Add there minced onion and garlic.
5. Add dried tomatoes and spinach.
6. Pour all the mixture into the Crock Pot, add Feta cheese.
7. Cover and cook on LOW 5-6 hours.
8. Bon Appetite!

Chapter 3: Lunch Recipes

Avocado Toad in the Hole

Such a cute name for a simple lunch. The first time when I heard the name of this recipe I thought that someone just mispronounces the word "toast" and that this recipe definitely has something to do with bread. But I stayed corrected and it turned to be a good thing, since eating avocados is healthier than eating bread. Moreover, it gives lots of healthy fats and vitamins to get you through the first half of the day with an egg-cellent mood.

Ingredients (6 servings):

avocados	3 medium pcs
eggs	6 medium
garlic powder	1 teaspoon
sea salt	1/2 teaspoon
black pepper	1/4 teaspoon
Parmesan cheese	1/4 cup

Directions:
1. Wash and cut in half avocados, remove the pits. Scoop out about 1/4 of the meat from each half. You must create enough space for the egg to fit inside.
2. Open the Crock Pot and spray the cooking spray over the bottom.
3. Place the avocado halves into the bottom of the Crock Pot.
4. Sprinkle each one with salt, garlic powder, and black pepper.
5. Grate the Parmesan cheese.
6. Crack a fresh egg into each half of the avocado and sprinkle with cheese.
7. Cover the Crock Pot and put on HIGH for 1 hour.
8. The egg whites must no longer jiggle.
9. Eat while still warm.
10. Bon Appetite!

Japanese Pumpkin Dip

Today we say «Hello» to this delicious and tasty Japanese pumpkin dip. And the best thing is that you don't even need to go to Japan or Thailand to taste this amazing and colorful dip. Everything you need to do is to follow my instructions, be patient and you will get a tasty, light dip for lunch!

Ingredients (11 servings):

Japanese pumpkin	3 lbs
olive oil	1/4 cup
sea salt	1 teaspoon
white onion	1 medium
unsalted butter (or ghee)	2 tablespoons
heavy cream (or coconut cream)	2 cups
garlic powder	1 tablespoon
sea salt	1 teaspoon
fresh rosemary	4 sprigs
water or broth	1/2 - 1 cup
pumpkin seeds	1/3 cup

Directions:
1. Wash the Japanese pumpkin and remove the seeds.
2. Chop into 2-inch cubes.
3. Open the Crock Pot and spray the cooking spray over the bottom.
4. Put the cubes onto the bottom of the Crock Pot, drizzle with olive oil and season with salt. Cover and put on HIGH for 2 hours.
5. Peel and chop finely the white onion, cook it until golden in a little saucepan with unsalted butter.

6. Once the onion is translucent, put it into a bowl. Set aside.
7. Whip heavy cream in a food processor for about 5 minutes.
8. Add the cooked onion, garlic powder, salt and fresh rosemary. Blend everything well.
9. Once the pumpkin is ready, let it cool a little bit and peel the skin off. Blend the peeled pumpkin in the food processor together with the whipped cream mixture until creamy.
10. Transfer the pumpkin soup into the Crock Pot and put on LOW for 1 more hour.
11. Serve with pumpkin seeds!
12. Enjoy warm!

Blackberry Egg Keto Bake

This recipe is perfect for those who are lazy but still like to enjoy something tasty and unusual. It requires very little time to make and is pretty delicious. This recipe includes an unusual flavor combination and the texture is fantastic. The rosemary, lime zest and ginger combined together with a little bit of vanilla give the eggs and the fresh blackberries an interesting twist.

Ingredients (9 servings):

eggs	5 large
butter (melted)	1 tablespoon

coconut flour	3 tablespoons
grated fresh ginger	1 teaspoon
vanilla	1/4 teaspoon
fine sea salt	1/3 teaspoon
zest of lime	1/2 tablespoon
fresh rosemary	1 teaspoon
fresh blackberries	1/2 cup

Directions:

1. Open the Crock Pot and spray the cooking spray over the bottom.
2. Melt the butter in a little saucepan.
3. Finely chop fresh rosemary.
4. Place freshly cracked eggs, melted butter, coconut flour, freshly grated ginger, vanilla, salt, zest into a blender and process for about two minutes on high. The mixture must be fully combined and smooth.
5. Add the rosemary and pulse for a few times until the rosemary is just incorporated.
6. Put the egg mixture into the Crock Pot, add the blackberries.
7. Cover the Crock Pot and set on HIGH for 1 hour, until the egg mixture puffs and is fully cooked through.
8. Let it cool for a few minutes once cooked. Add chopped rosemary.
9. Bon Appetite!

Quick Sausage Lunch for Two

Quick sausage lunch is great because you put all the ingredients in the Crock Pot and let it cook. Today I decided to combine the robust flavors of Italian sausages with full of carbs with species, ketchup, and veggies. A plenty of melted cheese will never damage your dish!

Ingredients (9 servings):

sausage	5 pcs
white onion	1 tablespoon
ketchup	1/2 cup
Parmesan cheese	1/4 cup
shredded mozzarella	1/4 cup
oregano	1/2 teaspoon
basil	1/2 teaspoon
salt	1/4 teaspoon
red pepper	1/4 teaspoon

Directions:

1. Open the Crock Pot and spray the cooking spray over the bottom.
2. Cut the sausages into rounds (about 1/2 inch) and put them to the Crock Pot.
3. Shred mozzarella and Parmesan cheese.
4. Peel and finely dice the onion. Add to the Crock Pot also.

5. Pour the ketchup and Parmesan cheese. Stir to combine everything well.
6. Add onion, oregano, pepper, and salt. Cover the Crock Pot and set on LOW for 2 – 3 hours.
7. Once the cooking time is over, open the Crock Pot and sprinkle with mozzarella cheese.
8. Sprinkle with basil.
9. Bon Appetite!

Shakshuka Keto Crock Pot

This dish can be enjoyed together with all your family and friends or you may eat it alone. It's essentially a sauce made of tomatoes and finely chopped chili peppers. If you are bored of the usual scrambled eggs prepared for lunches, this can be a great alternative. Enjoy preparing your sauce if you have a plenty of time and a really awesome recipe. This time I decided to use one of my favorite marinara sauces.

Ingredients (7 servings):

marinara sauce	1 cup
pepper	1 chili
eggs	4 pcs
feta cheese	1 oz
cumin	1/8 teaspoon

salt

pepper

fresh basil (at will)

or fresh oregano (if desired)

Directions:
1. Finely chop the chili. But be careful!
2. Take a medium-sized bowl and add a cup of marinara sauce, chopped chili. Whisk everything together
3. Crack fresh eggs to the marinara and chili mixture, continue whisking.
4. Crumble the feta cheese and sprinkle it over the marinara-eggs mix, season this with pepper and salt at will. Add cumin.
5. Open the Crock Pot and spray the cooking spray over the bottom.
6. Pour the mix into the Crock Pot, cover and set on LOW for 2 hours. Check the dish from time to time, it must seem not cooked enough rather to heat itself.
7. Once the time is over, the eggs must be still runny a little. Transfer the shakshuka from the Crock Pot on a plate carefully, helping with spoon or blade.
8. Wash and chop fresh basil, sprinkle it over the ready dish.
9. Enjoy!

Keto Feta & Pesto Omelet

This keto omelet is absolutely great for a season of fresh and flavor basil. This time pesto must be on the menu, of course, if you like it. That's why I decided to cook this quick Italian lunch and namely pesto and feta omelet. The end result I became after mixing all these simple and delicious ingredients was really great. I don't want even describe this sunny, delicate and herby pesto omelet but wish you cook it quickly.

Ingredients (5 servings):

Butter	1 tablespoon
Eggs	5 pcs
heavy cream	1 tablespoon
feta cheese	1 oz.
pesto	1 tablespoon
salt	
pepper	

Directions:

1. Take a medium-sized saucepan and heat it up. Melt a tablespoon of butter.
2. Take another little bowl, crack the fresh eggs, add melted butter and put a tablespoon of heavy cream. (If you want to get your omelet fluffy).

3. Open the Crock Pot and spray the cooking spray over the bottom.
4. Pour the eggs mix into the Crock Pot and put on LOW for 1-1,5 hours until fully cooked.
5. Once the time is almost over, open the Crock Pot and sprinkle pesto on the top of the dish.
6. Shred the feta cheese and spread it over the top of the omelet also.
7. Cover the Crock Pot and wait until the feta cheese is fully melted over the omelet.
8. Once the feta is melted, transfer the ready dish on a plate carefully and season with salt and pepper.
9. Garnish with more feta at will and fresh basil leaves if desired or cherry tomatoes.
10. Bon Appetite!

Egg Clouds & Bacon Weave

Have you ever tried the egg clouds? It is awesome! You just whisk them into a foamy peak and bake. When I firstly whisked the egg whites into foam I was rather skeptical as I could do this creation only using eggs and blender. I couldn't believe it happened so quick and so easy. The egg whites made a cloud-like creation that is a rather beautiful creation of mine. Finally, I added egg yolks that stayed rather fluffy inside. If you like to get bacon crispy, prebake the strips for about 7 minutes before you add the egg whites.

Ingredients (6 servings):

Bacon   6 – 9 strips

Eggs   2 pcs

Salt   1/2 teaspoon

garlic powder 1/2 tsp

pepper   1/4 teaspoon

cayenne   1/4 teaspoon

Directions :

1. Firstly, let's prepare the bacon waves: take three strips of bacon per cloud and fold them in half lengthwise. Ensure that both halves have the same length. They must create a perfect square bed.
2. Lay three long strips of bacon parallel to each other and fold the middle strip over. Put a strip perpendicular to the three, fold back over. Take the two outer strips and fold over.
3. Put another bacon strip in the center perpendicularly. Turn over the middle strip on the weave.
4. Put the final strip and tuck up. If you like to get bacon crispy, prebake the strips for about 6-7 minutes before you add the egg whites.
5. Take a medium-sized bowl, separate eggs and leave the yolks in a bowl. Do not break the yolks it is of high importance.

6. Put the egg whites in another deep bowl, whisk the egg whites with blender for about 7 minutes. The egg white must be thick, white foam.
7. Add salt and garlic powder and whisk all together. Be attentive, if you add these ingredients earlier, the eggs could take longer to form the cloudiness.
8. Open the Crock Pot and spread the cooking spray on a bottom and sides of the Crock Pot.
9. Place the bacon waves on the bottom of the Crock Pot, using a spoon place your seasoned egg whites onto the weave and create a little cloud.
10. Carefully make a little dip in a cloud (in each one) and place the egg yolk there.
11. Season the tops of the egg clouds with paprika and cayenne pepper.
12. Cover the Crock Pot and set on HIGH for 1 hour, until the egg clouds have become golden.
13. Once the time is over, transfer your creation carefully on a plate and sprinkle with some coarse salt!
14. Bon Appetite!

Avocado Fries Crock Pot

Have searched for amazing quick lunch recipes? You have found the recipe you must cook for sure! Simple to make, keto-friendly, quick and flavor!

Crispy outside and tender inside. Every beat of this tasty lunch is full of fat, so you will not feel hunger the rest of the day! If you don't like sriracha hot sauce, feel free to prepare the other one like garlic dip or cilantro lime dip.

Ingredients (8 servings):
Fries

Avocados	3 pcs
Egg	1 pcs
almond meal	1 1/2 cups
sunflower oil	1 1/2 cups
cayenne pepper	1/4 teaspoon
salt	1/2 teaspoon

Spicy Mayo

homemade mayo	2 tablespoon
sriracha	2 tablespoon

Directions:
1. Take a medium-sized bowl, crack a fresh egg into this bowl, whisk it thoroughly.
2. Tae another medium bowl, join the almond meal with a little bit salt and cayenne pepper.
3. Wash and slice avocados in half, carefully take out the seeds.
4. Peel off the skin off every half.

5. Slice each slice of avocado 4 or 5 pieces (if it is rather big).
6. Open the Crock Pot and sunflower oil to the bottom of the Crock Pot.
7. Coat each of avocado slices the egg mixture.
8. Put each avocado slice in the almond meal carefully, do this until you will not fully see the avocado green.
9. Place each covered slice of avocado into the Crock Pot.
10. Cover and put on HIGH for 2 hours. Turn the slices from time to time.
11. Once the cooking time is over, transfer slices quickly to a plate.
12. In a little bowl, mix sriracha sauce and mayo and deep the avocado slices before eating!
13. Enjoy hot!

Spicy Shrimp Omelet Crock Pot

This healthy and quick lunch idea is easy to cook and amazing to eat. If you have never tried shrimp in the omelet or with eggs, I think this recipe will be great for opening new tastes. I was very pleased with the result I got finally.

Ingredients (8 servings):

Shrimp   10 large

Eggs   6 pcs

grape tomatoes	4 pcs
spinach	1 handful
onion	1/4
sriracha salt	1 tablespoon
parsley	1 sprig
cayenne	1/4 teaspoon

Directions:

1. Peel and chop the onion.
2. Take a medium-sized saucepan, put it over medium heat and place onions. Season this with salt. Cook for some minutes.
3. Wash and slice the tomatoes in half lengthwise.
4. Add the grape tomatoes to onions and, cut side down and cook a little.
5. Wash and chop the spinach.
6. Once the onions are translucent, add spinach and let it cook for some minutes.
7. Open the Crock Pot and pour the mix of tomatoes, onions, and spinach into the Crock Pot. Add cayenne. Cover and put on HIGH for 2 hours.
8. Add shrimp and brake fresh eggs. If you wish to whisk them for a little.
9. Once the omelet is ready, transfer your dish on a plate!
10. Garnish with some parsley and enjoy!
11. Bon Appetite!

Keto Crock Pot lunch balls

I know a lot of people who prefer to have essential lunch during their busy working day. I think this recipe of the quick and essential meatballs it that recipe they could look for. Lunch balls are great in a combination of caramelized onions. It is something like a burger if you eat this with keto bread.

Ingredients (15 servings):

ground beef	1/2 lb
bacon	1 strip
jalapenos	1 tablespoon
mayo	1 tablespoon
tomato	1/2 plum
onion	¼ pcs
sriracha	1 tablespoon
egg	1 pcs
butter	2 tablespoon
lettuce	2 leaves

Spices

Salt	1/2 teaspoon
crushed red pepper	1/2 teaspoon
cayenne	1/4 teaspoon

basil   1/2 teaspoon

Directions:
1. Knead the meat for about 4-5 minutes. This makes it sticky and keeps it together when you add all the ingredients to it.
2. Chop the bacon.
3. Chop finely jalapenos. Crush the red peppers.
4. Wash and slice tomatoes. Pell the onion and cut.
5. Take a large bowl, combine the onion, mayo, sriracha, freshly cracked egg, salt, red pepper, basil, and cayenne. Stir everything well. Add this to the ground beef. Knead it again once more.
6. Make balls from the meat.
7. Open the Crock Pot, sprinkle the bottom with oil or ghee.
8. Put the meatballs on the bottom.
9. Cover and put on HIGH for 3 hours. Turn balls from time to time.
10. Once the dish is ready, combine it with caramelized onions.
11. Bon Appetite!

Healthy Spaghetti Squash

This recipe of the dish doesn't have to be rather exact. I would say, you may add also other ingredients to the spaghetti squash. Add another kind of cheese or another mix of veggies. Make your own breakfast!

Ingredients (8 servings):

spaghetti squash	1 pcs
salt and pepper at will	
tomato sauce	2 - 3 tablespoon
spinach	1 - 2 handfuls
ham	2 slices
red onion	1 - 2 thin slices
Cheddar cheese	1 handful
green onions	1 handful
eggs	2 pcs

Directions:
1. Wash and chop the spinach. Set aside.
2. Chop the ham into slices.
3. Peel the onion and slice the onion.
4. Shred the Cheddar cheese. Set aside.
5. Chop the green onions.
6. Wash and slice the squash in half, take off the seeds.
7. Sprinkle the squash with pepper and salt to taste.
8. Spread a little bit tomato sauce into the squash.
9. Put the spinach, cheese, ham, red onion.

10. Open the Crock Pot and spray with cooking
    spray the bottoms and the sides.
11. Put the filled spaghetti squash in the Crock Pot.
12. Crack two eggs into the spaghetti squash.
    Cover the lid and set on HIGH for 4 hours.
13. Once the time is over, dress with pepper and
    salt.
14. Serve warm.
15. Bon Appetite!

Chapter 4: Seafood Recipes

Cajun Crab Keto Crock Pot

A tasty and quick keto cajun crab dish with delicious seasoning is perfect for both breakfast, dinner and even supper. If you don't prefer celery stalks you may don't use them at all or add other veggies – onions, basil leaves etc. Enjoy warm!

Ingredients (11 servings):

Butter	1 oz.
yellow onion	1 pcs
celery stalks	5 1/3 oz.
mayonnaise	1¼ cups
eggs	4 pcs freshly
shredded cheese	2/3 lb
crab meat (120 g/can be drained)	1 lb canned
paprika powder	2 teaspoons

| cayenne pepper | ¼ teaspoon |
| salt and pepper | |

For serving

| leafy greens | 3 oz. |
| olive oil | 2 tablespoons |

Directions:
1. Peel and chop the onion and celery finely.
2. Take a medium-sized saucepan, add butter and roast a little onion and celery until translucent. Dress with salt and pepper at will.
3. Shred the cheese and set aside.
4. Take another deep bowl, add mayo, freshly cracked eggs, crab meat, seasonings and ⅔ of the shredded cheese.
5. Add the fried onion and celery. Mix everything well and season at will.
6. Open the Crock Pot and spray with the cooking spray finely. Pour the mix into the Crock Pot.
7. Add the remaining cheese on top and on LOW for 3 hours until golden brown.
8. Serve with salad and black pepper!
9. Bon Appetite!

Keto Smoked Mussels Crock Pot

Have a busy weekend but still want to cook some delicious? Canned seafood to the rescue! Take a bowl and combine smoked mussels with cheese and cauliflower, and have a perfect keto dinner on the table in half an hour.

Ingredients (9 servings):

Cauliflower	1 lb
yellow onion	½ pcs
Dijon mustard	2 tablespoons
Mayonnaise	1 cup
shredded cheddar cheese	7 oz.
fresh chives (optional)	2 tablespoons
mussels	10 oz. canned
salt and pepper	

Serving

Lettuce	4¼ oz.
olive oil	4 tablespoons

Directions:
1. Wash and cut the cauliflower into small florets and put them in a pot.
2. Add water, it must cover the florets.
3. Add salt and bring to a boil. Let the cauliflower boil for a couple of minutes.
4. Drain the cauliflower and discard the water.
5. Peel the onion and chop the onion finely.
6. Shred the cheddar cheese. Set aside.

7. Take a deep bowl, put the onion, mustard, mayo and ⅔ parts of the cheese in a bowl and mix everything well.
8. Open the Crock Pot, pour the mixture, add cauliflower and mussels.
9. Cover and put on LOW for 3 hours.
10. Once the dish is ready, sprinkle the remaining grated cheese on top and set on WARM.
11. Serve with lettuce.
12. Bon Appetite!

Broiled Sea Bass with Chili Basil Glaze

Seabass with basil-chili glaze tastes super tender and amazing. You may serve this dish with cauliflower rice or noodles, fresh veggies or anything you like but that correspond the ketogenic diet. You don't need to much time, just to wash the filets, sprinkle with species. The other part of work will do the Crock Pot.

Ingredients (7 servings):

Vinegar	2 tablespoons
chopped basil	1 teaspoon
red pepper	1/8 teaspoon
garlic	1 clove
salt, divided	3/4 teaspoon

sea bass fillet   4 (6-ounce)

black pepper   1/4 teaspoon

Cooking spray

Directions:
1. Wash the fish fillet and dry it with a paper towel.
2. Peel the garlic and mince.
3. Wash fresh basil, chop finely.
4. Crush the red pepper. Set aside.
5. Open the Crock Pot, spray with cooking spray the bottom and sides of it.
6. Take a medium bowl, conjoin vinegar, basil, red pepper, garlic, salt.
7. Season the fillets with salt and black pepper at will.
8. Place the sea bass fillets on a bottom of the Crock Pot, sprinkle with species.
9. Cover the lid and put on HIGH for 4 hours or until the fillets are tender when tested with a fork.
10. Bon Appetite!

Crock Pot Keto Sea Bass

Cooking of the sea bass in a traditional way is of high importance to check the time. The sea bass must not be overcooked or undercooked, otherwise, the taste and the fish will be damaged. The time that is suggested at the recipe is the optimal period for cooking the fish tender but stay juicy.

Ingredients (5 servings):

sea bass	1 whole fish
sea salt	1 tsp
fresh dill	3 sprigs
fresh parsley	2 sprigs
lemon zest	
pepper at will	

Seasoning: 1 tsp sea salt + 2 tsp olive oil

Directions:
1. Shred the lemon zest in a plate. Set aside. Wash fresh parsley and dill.
2. Wash the fish thoroughly, rinse well. Take off the scales, wipe dry.
3. Season with sea salt from both sides - inside and outside of the sea bass.
4. Open the Crock Pot, spray with cooking spray the bottom and sides of it.
5. Put the whole fish on the bottom of the Crock Pot.
6. Dress the fish with sprigs of dill and parsley. Put the lemon zest over the fish. Drizzle a little with olive oil.

7. Cover the lid and put on HIGH for 3 hours, the sea bass must get tender when tested with a fork.
8. Remove the fish carefully from the Crock Pot once the cooking time is over and serve on a plate.
9. Serve hot.

Sea Bass with Fennel and Tomatoes

The tender taste of sea bass is combined with flavor tomatoes and fennel in this recipe… How delicious is it! You can't imagine. Check the tenderness of sea bass all the time while cooking it in the Crock Pot, it is of high importance cooking the fish in a right way. It is a super tasty combination of the Mediterranean classic ingredients.

Ingredients (11 servings):
Cooking the sea bass:

fillets of sea bass	6 oz
olive oil	1 tablespoon
salt and ground black pepper at will	

Cooking tomatoes and fennel:

fennel	4 bulbs
extra virgin olive oil	6 fl oz

tomatoes	1 big can
garlic	1 head
boiling water	5 fl oz
dry white wine	120ml/4fl oz
chopped fresh oregano leaves	2 tablespoon
balsamic vinegar	2 tablespoon
basil leaves	12 pcs

Directions:

1. Wash the fish thoroughly, rinse well. Take off the scales, wipe dry. Take off the skin. Place the pieces in the fridge.
2. Peel the garlic and mince. Wash the fresh leaves of oregano and chop.
3. Remove leaves from fennel.
4. Cut the fennel lengthways into quarters.
5. Heat the oil in a medium-sized saucepan and put the fennel. Cook the fennel turning frequently, for 15 minutes. Fennel must be of brown color.
6. Add the chopped tomatoes, minced garlic, boiling water, wine, oregano and black pepper at will.
7. Let the mixture boil, cover the lid of the saucepan and cook for 20 minutes.
8. Once the ingredients are almost cooked, add balsamic vinegar and basil leaves. Cover with lid again.

9. Take the sea bass from the refrigerator, season with salt and pepper.
10. Open the Crock Pot, spray with cooking spray the bottom and sides of it.
11. Place the sea bass on a bottom of the Crock Pot.
12. Cover the lid and put on HIGH for 4 hours or until the fish is tender when tested with a fork.
13. Remove the fish carefully from the Crock Pot once the cooking time is over and serve on a plate.
14. Place with a spoonful of the tomatoes and fennel into the center of each piece of fish.
15. Enjoy warm!

Keto Sea Bass Cuban Style

This recipe of the sea bass fish fillets is easy to cook and sure to please! This one is great for parties, guests, friends and you don't need special time (if you don't have it at all) to be present all the day long at the kitchen.

Ingredients (9 servings):

olive oil	2 teaspoon
white onions	1 1/2 cups
minced garlic	2 teaspoon
fresh tomatoes	4 cups

dry white wine	1 1/2 cups
red pepper flakes	1/8 teaspoon
fillets sea bass	4 (6 ounces)
butter	2 teaspoon
fresh cilantro	1/4 cup

Pepper and salt at will

Directions:

1. Peel the onion and chop. Peel the garlic and mince finely. Wash and chop fresh cilantro. Set aside.
2. Wash the tomatoes, dry with paper towel, take off the seeds, chop them.
3. Heat olive oil in a medium saucepan over high heat. Sautee onions for some time until it gets brown color. Add garlic, and saute for minutes.
4. Add tomatoes. They must begin to soften.
5. Add wine, toss and add red pepper flakes. Let everything boil a little bit. Add butter. The sauce must thicken.
6. Open the Crock Pot, spray with cooking spray the bottom and sides of it.
7. Place the sea bass fillets on a bottom of the Crock Pot. Pour the sauce over the fillets.
8. Cover the lid and put on LOW for 6 hours or until the fish is tender when tested with a fork. But check the tenderness of fish fillets from time to time they must not be overcooked.

9. Remove the fish carefully from the Crock Pot
    once the cooking time is over and serve on a
    plate together with sauce from the Crock Pot.
10. Serve with fresh dill or cilantro at will.
11. Bon Appetite!

Keto Sticky Asian Sea Bass

I like this recipe for Asian sea bass very much.
Delicate and a little bit soft, but it is still totally
versatile. It tastes delicious. Take off the skin from the
fillets, prepare the sweet-soy sauce that is a perfect
adding to your fish and wait until the Crock Pot will
cook the fish fillets for you. Add to the fish chili and
coriander. It is perfectly well!

Ingredients (9 servings):

sesame oil	1 tablespoon
red chili	½ pcs
sweetener	3 tablespoon
dark soy sauce replaces with tamari	1 tablespoon
ground ginger	1/4 teaspoon
garlic	1 clove
Juice of lime	¼ of a lime
Sea Bass fillets - skin on	2 fillets

Almond flour   ½ teaspoon

fresh coriander torn

pepper and salt at will

Directions:
1. Peel the garlic and mince finely.
2. Take off the skin of the sea bass fillets.
3. Take a medium-sized bowl, mix the oil, chili, sweetener, soy sauce, ginger, minced garlic.
4. Squeeze the juice of a lime and add to the mixture.
5. Open the Crock Pot, spray with cooking spray the bottom and sides of it.
6. Place the sea bass fillets on a bottom of the Crock Pot.
7. Sprinkle with the flour.
8. Sprinkle with sweet-soy sauce mix.
9. Cover the lid and put on LOW for 6 hours or until the fish is tender when tested with a fork.
10. Once the cooking time is over, remove the fillets from the Crock Pot on a plate and sprinkle with remained sauce, season with coriander and chili slices.
11. Enjoy warm.

Healthy Crock Pot Fish Fillet

I think every person is going to eat only healthy organic food. What could be healthier than to consume fish that is full of microelements and vitamins? To prepare the fish fillets following this recipe you may choose almost any fish you prefer most and mix with favorite species. Add lemon slices to get the tender taste of the fish and to avoid the smell.

Ingredients (5 servings):

salt, or to taste   1 teaspoon

fresh ground black pepper   1/2 teaspoon

white fish (cod, sea bass or catfish)   2-3 lb

fresh herbs (mix of parsley, basil, savory, tarragon)

lemons   2-3 pcs

Directions:
1. Wash and dry with paper towel lemons. Slice thinly. Set aside.
2. Wash the fish thoroughly, rinse well. Take off the scales, wipe dry. Take off the skin.
3. Sprinkle all the sides of the fish with pepper and salt.
4. Open the Crock Pot, spray with cooking spray the bottom and sides of it.
5. Place the fillets on a bottom of the Crock Pot.
6. Place the lemon slices and herbs on top of the fish.

7. Cover the Crock Pot and put on HIGH for 4-5 hours (depending on the fish) until the fish is cooked through fully.
8. Once the cooking time is over, remove the lemon slices and serve the fish fillet with your favorite species.
9. Bon appetite!

Crock Pot Tuna Mornay

This tuna Mornay is super easy and tender. Everything you need is to buy a can of tuna, add your favorite cheese (Parmesan or Cheddar, as for me), add sour cream and celery soup and wait for tasty dinner!

Ingredients (6 servings):

condensed cream of celery soup	1 can
tuna, with brine (with liquid)	1 425g can
sour cream	½ cup
shallots	3 pcs
water	1/3 cup
Parmesan or cheddar cheese	1 cup

salt and pepper at will

Directions:
1. Pell and chop the shallots.

2. Take a medium-sized bowl, join the condensed cream of celery soup, tuna, sour cream, water, shallots. Add also the rest liquid from the tuna.
3. Open the Crock Pot, put all the mixture, cover the lid of the Crock Pot and put on LOW for 4 hours.
4. Once the cooking time is over, open the lid, add shredded cheese and cover for 30 minutes.
5. Serve hot.
6. Bon Appetite!

Crock Pot Fillet of Sole with Pesto

This amazing recipe needs only three main ingredients! Could you imagine this?! You need only fish fillets, pesto, and shredded cheese. I don't recommend to add the water as the fish fillets could be overcooked. When the fillets are done they are of white color and tender, check this using a fork.

Ingredients (3 servings):

white fish (sole)	1 to 2 pounds
bottled pesto	1 bottle
shredded Parmesan cheese	½ cups
salt and pepper at will	
mint for dressing	

Directions:

1. Shred the Parmesan cheese. Set aside.
2. Wash the fish thoroughly, rinse well. Take off the scales, wipe dry. Take off the skin.
3. Open the Crock Pot, spray with cooking spray the bottom and sides of it.
4. Place the fillets on a bottom of the Crock Pot.
5. Cover the sole fillets with pesto (1-2 spoons on each fillet).
6. Sprinkle with shredded Parmesan each piece of sole.
7. Cover the lid and put on LOW for 4 hours.
8. Once the cooking time is over, open the Crock Pot and remove the ready-made fish fillets on a plate.
9. You may serve the fish fillets with veggies like spinach, zucchini, asparagus etc.
10. Eat warm. Serve with fresh mint.
11. Bon Appetite!

Sole in Herbed Butter

This recipe was advised me many years ago by my old friend. Since that time I have prepared this dish many times as it is simple and quick. Dill and lemon is the best mix of herbed butter and sole. Don't hesitate to cook it today!

Ingredients (7 servings):

Butter   4 teaspoon

dill weed	1 teaspoon
onion powder	1/2 teaspoon
garlic powder	1/2 teaspoon
salt	1/2 teaspoon
white pepper	1/4 teaspoon
sole fillets	2 pounds

Fresh dill and lemon wedges for dressing

Directions:
1. Wash the fish thoroughly, rinse well. Take off the scales, wipe dry. Take off the skin.
2. Take a medium-sized bowl, conjoin the butter, onion powder, dill, garlic powder, salt at will and pepper if desired.
3. Open the Crock Pot, spray with cooking spray the bottom and sides of it.
4. Add the sole on a bottom of the Crock Pot and put the herbed mixture over each fish fillet.
5. Garnish with lemon and dill if desired.
6. Cover the lid and put on LOW for 5 hours.
7. Once the cooking time is over, open the Crock Pot and take off the fish fillets on a serving plate.
8. Bon Appetite!

Jamaican salmon Crock Pot recipe

Preparing the salmon according to this recipe you may mix all the species that are mentioned below or just buy the mix of species in a store. As for me, I Like to use my handmade species because I know what I want to mix and the ingredients are always fresh. I advise you to follow strictly my instructions. Don't open the foil packet during the cooking time, otherwise, the juice from fish will flow out.

Ingredients (11 servings):

Cloves	1/8 teaspoon
Ginger	1/8 teaspoon
Nutmeg	1/8 teaspoon
kosher salt	1 teaspoon
onion powder	1 teaspoon
sweetener	2 teaspoons
chipotle chili powder	1/4 teaspoon
cayenne pepper	1/2 teaspoon
black pepper	1/4 teaspoon
thyme	1/8 teaspoon
cinnamon	1/2 teaspoon

Directions:

1. Peel the garlic and mince finely.

2. Mix in a medium-sized bowl garlic minced,
    ginger, nutmeg, salt and pepper, onion powder,
    sweetener, chili powder, cayenne pepper,
    cinnamon.
3. Open the Crock Pot, spray with cooking spray
    the bottom and sides of it.
4. Put the fish on of foil in the middle. Season all
    sides of the fish with mix once more. Make an
    enclosed packet from the foil, the fish juice
    must stay inside.
5. Put the foil into the Crock Pot. Be attentive! Do
    not add water.
6. Cover the lid and cook on LOW for 3 hours.
    Don't open the foil until the finish of the cooking
    time.
7. Serve hot on a large plate (without foil) with
    fresh veggies!
8. Bon Appetite!

Clam chowder Crock Pot

This is the recipe for the clam chowder from
England! This amazing dish with a creamy texture is
perfect and light for sunny days. I usually serve it with
salad or keto bread. My family likes seafood prepared
in the Crock Pot very much. You may serve the clam
chowder with chopped fresh parsley or bacon slices.
I'm sure the seafood fans would like this creamy soup
very much!

Ingredients (11 servings):

Onion	1 pcs large
clams	3 cans (ca. 6.5 ounces each)
clam juice	8 ounces
dried thyme	1/2 teaspoon
salt or at will	1/4 teaspoon
pepper or at will	1/4 teaspoon
butter	2 tablespoons
almond flour	3 tablespoons
half and half	1 cup
whole milk	1 cup
bacon	2 slices chopped

parsley for garnish

Directions:
1. Peel one large onion and dice it. Set aside.
2. Chop the clams finely. Slice the bacon.
3. Spread the bottom of the Crock Pot with cooking spray, add there diced onion.
4. After this, add there two full cans of clams (with juice) and also one without it.
5. Pour one bottle of clam juice, add pepper, dried thyme, salt in the Crock Pot. Mix everything well.

6. Cover the Crock Pot and cook on HIGH for 3-4 hours.
7. Take a large bowl, place it on high heat and melt the butter there. Add almond flour.
8. Toss the mixture until the smooth consistency. Pour slowly half and half and milk. Continue to stir until thickened.
9. Pour this mixture into the Crock Pot, cover and continue to cook for an hour on LOW.
10. Serve warm, add sliced bacon strips and parsley.
11. Bon Appetite!

Chapter 5: Beef and Chicken Recipes

Crock Pot Keto BBQ Chicken Legs

What can you add to the recipe for BBQ chicken legs? – Everything! Everything you wish! BBQ chicken legs recipe is one of the eldest classic versions of the cooking the chicken legs! So tasty as nowhere else. I like hot sauces and eat them well. If you don't like the hot sauces or chili like me, you may reduce the proposed amounts.

Ingredients (8 servings):

chicken legs	2 lb(s)
BBQ sauce	1 ½ cup
cider vinegar	¼ cup
onion	1 medium
garlic	3 clove
Chili powder	1 tablespoon
Paprika	2 teaspoon

mustard powder   1 teaspoon

Worcestershire sauce

pepper and salt to taste

Directions:
1. Peel the onion, garlic, chop them finely.
2. Put the chicken legs to the Crock Pot, add chopped garlic and onion, pour the sauce and vinegar, stir together.
3. Add also paprika, mustard as well as chili powder, Worcestershire sauce, salt.
4. Combine everything thoroughly.
5. Cover and cook on LOW 6 hours.
6. Serve with cauliflower rice.
7. Bon Appetite!

Keto Whole Chicken in a Hot Sauce

This recipe of whole chicken in a hot sauce prepared in the Crock Pot is tender and moist. Once the whole chicken is ready, I remove it to the big plate, shred it in pieces take off the remained liquid and add the prepared hot sauce. Remove the skin of the chicken and let the rest of the chicken juice run out... You don't need to cook the other additional dishes (like cauliflower rice or etc.) and other seasonings. It is perfectly well. Enjoy it!

Ingredients (16 servings):

sweet paprika	2 ½ teaspoon
garlic powder	1 ½ teaspoon
freshly ground pepper	1 ½ teaspoon
coriander	½ teaspoon
caraway	½ teaspoon
whole chicken	1 4- to 5-lb

Hot Sauce

Ketchup	1 cup
vinegar	¼ cup
sweetener	½ cup
mustard	2 tablespoon
sea salt	1 teaspoon
chili powder	1 teaspoon
onion powder	1 teaspoon
garlic powder	¾ teaspoon
cayenne	¼ teaspoon
ground pepper	¼ teaspoon

Directions:

1. Spread the cooking spray over the bottom and sides of the Crock Pot.

2. Wash the chicken, take off the insides. Take a middle pan and join there garlic powder, salt, caraway, coriander, and paprika.
3. Put the chicken into the Crock Pot and add this mixture on the top of it. Thoroughly spread this along with the chicken. Be sure that both sides are perfectly covered with mixture.
4. Over cover and put on LOW for 8 hours. Check readiness of the whole chicken with a fork.

Preparing for a hot sauce

1. While the chicken is prepared in the Crock Pot, make ready the hot sauce: join the ketchup, vinegar, mustard, salt, chili powder, onion powder, garlic powder, cayenne and pepper in a bowl. Stir everything well. Let the mixture boil, add the sweetener, stir once more.
2. When the chicken is almost cooked (once the time is over), take off the liquid from the Crock Pot, pour the sauce with a hot sauce, over cover and put on WARM. Leave it in the Crock Pot for 1 hour.
3. Serve additionally with hot sauce. Eat warm.
4. Bon Appetite!

Crock Pot Keto Butter Chicken

Today I would like to introduce you a healthy and light version of classic Indian chicken. This tender chicken is rich in fragrant species and creamy sauce consistency, garam masala and curry powder make the base of the classic Indian version. To keep the sauce flavor and creamy I usually add to the sauce heavy cream and tomato paste. This fragrant dish challenges the best flavors of India, keeping your chicken thighs with full of juice.

Ingredients (14 servings):

almond flour	3 tablespoon
garam masala	1 tablespoon
ground cumin	1 teaspoon
curry powder	1 teaspoon
chicken thighs	3 lb(s)
cashews	½ cup
onion	1 pcs
garlic	4 cloves
jalapeno pepper	1 pcs
fresh ginger	1 tablespoon
tomatoes	2 pcs
heavy cream	¾ cup
tomato paste	2 tablespoon
Greek yogurt	¾ cup

Cilantro leaves at will

Salt and pepper

Directions:
1. Prepare the thighs – remove skin and bones from the chicken thighs. Cut each of them into 4 -5 pieces.
2. Peel the onion and garlic, chop them plenty.
3. Wash and dry with a paper towel the peppers. Remove the seeds, slice. Chop fresh ginger.
4. Wash the tomatoes, take off the seeds, slice or quarter them.
5. Take a little pan, join flour, species. Stir finely. Toss chicken thighs with flour mixture.
6. Grind the cashews in a blender.
7. Put the chicken thighs in the Crock Pot, add there masala, cumin, curry, nuts, peppers, onions and garlic, grated ginger, sliced tomatoes and tomato paste, heavy cream. Toss everything.
8. Dress additional with salt and pepper.
9. Cover and put on LOW for 5 hours.
10. Dress with cilantro. Add Greek yogurt at will.
11. Bon Appetite!

Crock Pot Thai Curry Chicken

This delicious recipe was introduced me some years ago by my old friend. I'm sure this recipe should be definitely included in your cookbook. The base of this amazing dish is the Thai sauce cooked from coconut milk, curry paste, sauce, ginger, peanut butter, garlic, lime, a sweetener that makes this sauce at the same time both sour and sweet. The contradiction of the tastes is amazing. Don't be confused when you read lime and sweetener in this recipe, the chicken is perfectly tasty. Be sure, you'll surprise your guests with a rainbow of tastes!

Ingredients (13 servings):

peanut butter	⅓ cup
light coconut milk	14 oz
sauce (your favorite one)	3 tablespoon
ginger (from a jar)	1 tablespoon
garlic (from a jar)	2 teaspoon
red curry paste	1 tablespoon
onion	1 pcs
sweetener	2 tablespoon
lime juice	1 pcs
red pepper (optional)	1 pcs
fresh cilantro	½ cup
chicken breasts	4 pcs
mussels sized (7 oz)	10 pcs medium

Directions:

1. Take a medium pan, combine there peanut butter, spicy sauce (your favorite one), ginger, coconut milk, ginger from a jar, lime juice, curry paste, sweetener. Stir everything and put this paste into the center of the Crock Pot. Wash red pepper, dry it with a paper towel, remove the seeds and slice. Set it aside.
2. Peel the onion and chop it, add to the Crock Pot also.
3. Wash and dry with a paper towel the chicken breasts. Cut them into pieces and add to the Crock Pot also.
4. Cover and cook 4 hours on LOW.
5. Once the chicken is ready remove it to the plate, add mussels with liquid, fresh chopped cilantro, and sliced pepper.
6. Dress with black pepper at will.
7. Bon Appetite!

Crock Pot Creamy Chicken and Veggies

For this recipe, you need only chicken thighs and broccoli, cauliflower as for the veggies. Once the dish is ready, you need just to mix the juice of the chicken, lemon juice, and cream cheese! You can't even imagine how easy, tasty and delicious is the texture! It is a luscious sauce. You'd better eat this creamy chicken and veggies with eggs noodles. Don't hesitate to go to the kitchen and follow the directions you may find below.

Ingredients (11 servings):

olive oil	1 teaspoon
chicken thighs	6 pcs (about 1½-2 pounds)
salt	¼ teaspoon
black pepper	¼ teaspoon
cauliflower florets	1 pound
broccoli florets	1 pound
oregano	1 teaspoon
garlic powder	½ teaspoon
lemon	1 pcs
cream cheese	4 ounces
lemon juice	1 teaspoon

Directions:
1. Wash and chop the fresh parsley. Set aside. Slice the lemon into ¼ inch slices.
2. Scale the skin and bones from the chicken thighs.
3. Spread the olive oil on the bottom and side of the Crock Pot. Put the chicken thighs on the bottom.

4. Season with pepper and salt. Top the florets of the broccoli and cauliflower on the chicken pieces.
5. Add garlic powder and oregano. Top the lemon slice over the florets.
6. Cover and put on LOW for 5 hours. Check the tenderness with a fork.
7. Remove lemon slices at the end of cooking time. Remove firstly the florets of broccoli and cauliflower, then chicken pieces and the rest of liquid.
8. Add the cream cheese and the lemon juice into a small pan, add also the remained juice of chicken from the Crock Pot and stir everything well.
9. Pour this cream cheese over the chicken pieces that are already on your plate.
10. Serve warm and enjoy!

Whole Tuscan Chicken Crock Pot

I must say, I love my Crock Pot very much. It is my right arm in the kitchen. I can't imagine how I could cook my favorite recipes without it!? Tuscan chicken prepared in the Crock Pot is something amazing and appetizing for me and whole my family. Everything I need here it is just to prepare the seasoning mix, wash the chicken, remove the insides, make a «massage» to the chicken using the readymade seasoning mix and that's all! The remained work is for my right arm. It cooks Tuscan chicken super tasty! I like to enjoy this chicken with fresh tomatoes and cucumbers. Let's try to cook a whole chicken in a Tuscan-style!

Ingredients (13 servings):

Salt	3 teaspoons
Paprika	2 teaspoons
thyme	1½ teaspoons
garlic salt	½ teaspoon
rosemary	½ teaspoon
oregano	¼ teaspoon
ground black pepper	¼ teaspoon
lemon (zest and juice from it)	1 pcs
garlic	8 cloves
onion	1 pcs
olive oil	2 tablespoons
whole chicken	3½ to 4½ pounds
lemon	1 pcs

Directions:
1. Take a middle pan and mix together salt, paprika, thyme, garlic salt, oregano, rosemary, black pepper. Set aside.

2. Peel the onion and chop. Peel garlic and mince it (or press). Wash the lemon and slice.
3. Grate the lemon zest and add to the mixture. Add also minced garlic and combine everything once more.
4. Put the chopped onions in the Crock Pot, squeeze the lemon juice into the Crock Pot at once, add also one spoon of olive oil to the onions and garlic in the Crock Pot.
5. Wash the chicken, dry with a paper towel. Take off the insides, fold-down the wings. Place the readymade seasonings on the chicken and worm. Add the remained olive oil, add also the seasoning inside the chicken. Place the chicken in the Crock Pot.
6. Cover and cook on LOW for 9 hours.
7. Serve the cooked chicken on a large plate together with veggies from the Crock Pot.
8. Bon Appetite!

Crock Pot Chicken with 40 Garlic Cloves

If you are a fan of garlic and chicken but haven't ever tasted chicken with garlic cloves, you have been really missing out. But! You are on the right side of the post if you are reading this recipe. Everything you need here – to buy garlic, some species, chicken legs. The hardest work here is… to peel the 40 garlic cloves! Yes, it is really complicated a little bit. But don't be scared of this work, the result worth it! It is a rather comforting dish at any time of the year!

Ingredients (7 servings):

chicken legs	10-12 pcs
garlic	40 cloves
onion	1 small
fresh lemon juice	2 tablespoons
thyme	4 sprigs
bay leaves	2 pcs
paprika	2 teaspoons

Salt and pepper

Directions:
1. Peel all the garlic cloves. Peel the onion and slice thinly.
2. Squeeze the lemon juice into a cup.
3. Spread the cooking spray of the Crock Pot, add on the bottom of it the half of the onion and a half of the garlic cloves.
4. Wash the chicken legs, season them with paprika, salt, pepper, place them over the onion-garlic bed.
5. Top with bay leaves and thyme. Add the remained onion and another half of the garlic cloves.

6. Add the chicken legs again, the remained thyme.
7. Spread the lemon juice over the dish. Cover and cook 7 hours.
8. Bon Appetite!

Crock Pot Creamy Buffalo Chicken

The creamy Buffalo chicken cooked at the Crock Pot tastes tender and amazing. It is so easy to prepare! This recipe must be a crowd pleaser, delicious and remarkably simple. I don't know somebody, who dislikes this recipe of the creamy chicken. Let the chicken pieces be cooked until the chicken parts fall apart. Add the cream cheese at the end of cooking time as well as the bounding mixture of flour and water. Enjoy each piece of this creamy chicken.

Ingredients (13 servings):

chicken breast	2 pounds
salt	½ teaspoon
Buffalo wing sauce	½ cup
chicken broth	½ cup
sweet onion	½ cup
celery	½ cup (about 2 ribs)
almond flour	¼ cup

water	3-4 tablespoons
cream cheese (softened)	1 (8 ounces) package
dried parsley flakes	¼ teaspoon
dried dill	¼ teaspoon
garlic powder	¼ teaspoon
onion powder	⅛ teaspoon
black pepper at will	

Directions:

1. Wash the chicken, dry it with a paper towel. Remove the bones and the skin. Cut into large pieces.
2. Peel the sweet onion and chop. Chop the celery.
3. Spread the pepper and salt over the chicken and put it into the Crock Pot.
4. Mix the Buffalo wing sauce with broth. Top the chicken with this mixture, chopped onions, and celery.
5. Cover and put on LOW for 6 hours. Check the chicken with a fork if it is tender.
6. While chicken is prepared, take a little pan, add flour with water, stir this to the Crock Pot at the end of the cooking time.
7. Take another little pan, combine here dill, parsley flakes, onion powder, garlic powder, cream cheese. Pour this into the Crock Pot also at the final of cooking time. Put on WARM.

8. Serve warm.
9. Bon Appetite

Keto Chicken and Sausage Mix

This recipe of keto chicken and sausage mix is indispensable in your daily life. What could be easier than to put chicken thighs into the Crock Pot, add there Italian or andouille sausages, stir with species that you prefer most of all and wait some hours until the Crock Pot cook this delicious addition to the veggies or cauliflower rice?

Ingredients (16 servings):

chicken thighs	8 pcs
sausages andouille or Italian	6 pcs
almond flour	½ cup
chicken broth	3 cups
tomatoes or boxed	26 ounces canned
yellow onion	1pcs
celery ribs	5 pcs
bell pepper	1 pcs
red bell pepper	1 pcs
garlic	4 cloves

dried oregano	1½ teaspoons
dried thyme	1½ teaspoons
smoked paprika	1½ teaspoons
salt	1 teaspoon
cayenne pepper	¾ teaspoons
black pepper	¼ teaspoon

Directions:

1. Peel the onion and chop. Chop the celery ribs. Peel the garlic and mince.
2. Wash and dry with a paper towel bell pepper. Slice it.
3. Wash the chicken thighs, remove the skin. Put them into the Crock Pot.
4. Cut the sausages (optional – you may fry them at the pan). Add them to the Crock Pot too.
5. Add chicken broth, almond flour, chopped tomatoes from a can, chopped celery, sliced pepper, onions, red pepper, oregano, garlic, thyme, salt, paprika, black and cayenne pepper.
6. Toss everything finely.
7. Cover and put on LOW for 6 hours.
8. Serve with cauliflower rice or your favorite veggies. Bon Appetite!

Crock Pot Chicken Cacciatore

What do you know about Italian chicken cacciatore? Cacciatore means a «hunter-style» dish cooked from chicken, tomatoes, onions, vegetables, vinegar. This is one of the recipes I have found many years ago. I have tried too many versions of Italian cacciatore, but this one is the best one. Following this name «hunter-style», I hunted at the nearest supermarket, bought all necessary ingredients and returned home with a spoil. Now, I invite you to prepare the real chicken cacciatore together with me. Let's try to do it!

Ingredients (15 servings):

sweet onion	1 large
chicken thighs	6 pcs (roughly 1¾-2 pounds)
bell peppers	3 pcs
garlic	8 cloves
tomato paste	2 ounces
roasted diced tomatoes with juice	2 (14½ ounce each) cans
small artichoke hearts	2 (14-ounce cans each)
chicken broth	1 cup
bay leaf	1 pcs

fresh parsley	2 teaspoons
red pepper	½ teaspoon
dried rosemary leaves	½ teaspoon
salt	½ teaspoon
ground black pepper	¼ teaspoon
fresh basil leaves	10 pcs

Directions:
1. Peel and slice the sweet onions. Wash and dry with a paper towel bell pepper. Slice them.
2. Peel and half the garlic.
3. Put the onions on the bottom of the Crock Pot. Put the chicken thighs, add on the top of the garlic, pepper slices, tomato paste, diced tomatoes, salt, artichokes without liquid.
4. Add ground black pepper, rosemary leaves, parsley, chicken broth, bay leaf.
5. Cover and put on LOW for 5 hours.
6. Serve with black pepper and fresh basil leaves. Remove the bay leaf before serving.
7. Bon Appetite!

Keto Raspberry-Chipotle Chicken Tacos

From my point of view, this recipe of the raspberry-chipotle chicken tacos prepared in the

Crock Pot is great for a crowded party. A delicious meal without a huge of ingredients and an impressive amount of hard work. What do you need more? When I have a crowd of guests I always try to use this recipe, it works great! My Crock Pot makes all possible work so, preparing this dish makes fun. The sweetness of raspberry gets a new taste to a habitual chicken. I like to add to the ready-made dish shredded cheese (I can't imagine the most part of the dishes without cheese!), slices of avocado, sour cream. It tastes great!

Ingredients (8 servings):

chicken breasts	2 pounds
raspberry	⅓ cup
peppers in adobo sauce (sugar-free)	2 chipotle
garlic	1 clove
adobo sauce (from chipotle peppers)	1 tablespoon
kosher salt	1 tablespoon
cumin	½ teaspoon
roasted tomatoes	1 (15 ounces) can

Salt and pepper

Optional: shredded cheese, cilantro, slices of avocado, sour cream.

Directions:
1. Prepare the chicken breasts, remove the skin and the bones. Wash them and cut into halves. Put the chicken breasts on the bottom of the Crock Pot.
2. Peel the garlic, mince it.
3. Take a little pan, mix there.
4. Raspberries, minced garlic, chipotle peppers, salt, adobo sauce, cumin, pepper, blend until smooth consistency.
5. Pour the mixture over the chicken breasts in the Crock Pot, add roasted tomatoes on the top together with juice.
6. Cover and put on LOW for hours.
7. Remove the chicken breasts once they are ready together with the sauce, shred the breasts with the knife. Before serving add shredded cheese, some slices of avocado, two tablespoons of sour cream and enjoy!
8. Bon Appetite!

Strawberry-Habanero Pulled Chicken

The main ingredient of this dish is sauce… Yes, the strawberry-habanero sauce. Maybe, you think, it sounds strange, but you must taste it. Habanero peppers combined with the strawberry puree create a flavored sauce for the tender chicken. I usually add avocado slices to this chicken, it adds the sour-sweet-hot combination of sauce and chicken. Don't be scared of habanero peppers, the Crock Pot does it best – during the preparation time the pepper brings its natural sweetness.

Ingredients (12 servings):

fresh or frozen strawberry purée	1 cup
onion	¼ small
garlic	2 cloves
pepper	1 habanero
Sweetener	1 tablespoon
vinegar	1 tablespoon
molasses	1 tablespoon
tomato paste	1 teaspoon
liquid smoke	½ teaspoon
salt	1 pinch
chicken breasts	1 pound
avocado, sliced (optional)	1 pcs

Directions:

1. Peel the onion and chop it finely. Peel the garlic and smash. Wash and dry with a paper towel

habanero pepper, mince it carefully. Wash and slice the avocado.

2. Take a medium pan, mix there strawberry puree, chopped onions, smashed garlic, minced pepper, salt, sweetener, vinegar, tomato paste, molasses, liquid smoke. Stir well everything.

3. Remove the skin and the bones from the chicken breasts, wash them thoroughly. Toss the chicken breasts in the mixture and place them into the Crock Pot.

4. Cover and cook on HIGH for 3-4 hours.

5. Remove the chicken, shred it, pour the sauce and add the avocado slices.

6. Bon Appetite!

Crock Pot Chicken Korma

Spicy and creamy chicken Korma is an old Indian dish that you can cook at home. Chicken Korma is usually served in the Indian restaurant's menu. But this is my Crock Pot version where I combine chicken and the species together and cook everything for 6 hours, after this I also add Greek yogurt to get the creamy light texture of the dish. Following the rules of a keto diet, you may serve it with cauliflower rice for your guests or with keto bread.

Ingredients:

Tomatoes	5 mediums (about 1½ pounds)
onions	2 medium
garlic	3 cloves
fresh ginger	1 tablespoon
curry powder	2 teaspoons
garam masala	2 teaspoons
salt	½ teaspoon
red pepper flakes	¼ teaspoon
chicken drumsticks	8 pcs
Greek yogurt	½ cup
cilantro	¼ cup

Directions:

1. Wash the tomatoes, dry them with a paper towel. Take off the seeds, cut into quarters. Chop the fresh cilantro into a little bowl. Set aside.
2. Peel the onion and chop; peel the garlic and mince. Grate the fresh ginger into a plate.
3. Put in the Crock Pot tomatoes, chopped onions, minced garlic, grated ginger, salt, curry powder, masala, pepper flakes. Mix everything well.

4. Add chicken drumsticks in the mixture at the Crock Pot and toss everything.
5. Cover and put on LOW for 6 hours until chicken is tender. Check it with a fork.
6. Remove the chicken drumsticks to the plate, separate the meat from the bones and skin and return it to the Crock Pot.
7. Pour Greek yogurt, dress with pepper and salt at will.
8. Serve with chopped cilantro.
9. Eat warm.
10. Bon Appetite!

Crock Pot Chicken and Asparagus

The simple Crock Pot chicken recipe with tender asparagus makes a fragrant meal for whole your family. If you don't like the cream of onion soup, you might change it with cream of celery soup. The frozen asparagus is also OK for this recipe. My friend has replaced some ingredients with cream of broccoli, it was also great. So, you can vary a little bit here. You will not stain the dish, be sure! I would better say, be free to adapt this recipe to the preferred ingredients of your family. If you need an extra color, add some tomatoes or basil leaves.

Ingredients (12 servings):
chicken breasts   1 1/2 pounds (about 4 to 6 halves)

chicken stock	1/2 cup
cream of onion soup	1 (10 1/2-ounce) can
tarragon	1/4 to 1/2 teaspoon
lemon pepper seasoning	1 teaspoon
salt	1/4 teaspoon
asparagus	1 bunch
almond flour	1 tablespoon
milk	1 tablespoon
black pepper	
toasted almonds (optional)	
grated or shredded Parmesan cheese (optional)	

Directions:
1. Wash the breasts, take off the skin. Cut them into pieces. Put into the bottom of the Crock Pot.
2. Take a medium pan, mix there condensed soup, broth, seasoning, tarragon. Blend everything well.
3. Add this mix on the top of the chicken, cover and put on LOW for 5 hours. Put there also pepper and salt if needed.
4. While the chicken is in the Crock Pot, cut the asparagus into a 1-inch length. Add them

almost at the end of the cooking time to the breasts.

5. Take a small pan, whisk there milk and flour, add this mixture to the Crock Pot also.
6. Continue cooking (put on WARM) for 1 hour. The asparagus must get tenderness.
7. Garnish the ready-made chicken with grated Parmesan cheese and toasted almonds optional.
8. Bon Appetite!

Crock Pot Cashew Chicken

This cookie of the cashew chicken prepared in the Crock Pot needs just 10 minutes of preparation and I think you could find these 10 minutes easily. It is a flavorful and super easy dish that doesn't need special ingredients that couldn't be found on the shelves of the supermarkets. Everything you need could be found at the nearest shop. Let's try to do it!

Ingredients (11 servings):

chicken thighs	2 lbs
almond flour	1/2 teaspoon
canola oil	1 tablespoon
hot sauce	1/4 cup
vinegar	2 tablespoon

ketchup	2 tablespoon
xanthan gum	1 tablespoon
garlic	1 clove
grated fresh ginger	1/2 teaspoon
red pepper flakes	1/4 teaspoon
cashews	1/2 cup

Green onions (optional, for garnish)

black pepper

Directions:
1. Peel the onion and mince. Grate the fresh ginger.
2. Chop green onions.
3. Prepare the chicken, take off the skin and the bones, cut into 6-7 pieces.
4. Take a storage bag, mix the flour with pepper flakes, add the chicken thighs. Shake the mixture and the chicken together. Chicken must be covered with the mixture.
5. Spread the cooking spray over the Crock Pot, put there coated chicken thighs.
6. Take another medium bowl, mix the vinegar, sauce, xanthan gum, minced garlic, pepper flakes (the rest of them), grated ginger, top over chicken.
7. Cover and put on LOW for 4 hours. Stir in the nuts and continue cooking 15 minutes more.

8. Serve hot! Add chopped green onions.

Chapter 6: Soups and Stews Recipes

Keto Pumpkin and Coconut Soup

Do you know the recipe how to prepare an easy keto coconut and pumpkin soup? Not yet? I will tell you the easiest and cheapest way to cook it. This soup prepared quickly in the Crock Pot is super winter warmer one! Moreover, you may freeze this tasty soup in small baking dishes (for example for baking of muffins in portions) and re-heat when you wish.

Ingredients (7 servings):

Yellow onion	1 pcs medium
ginger	1 teaspoon
garlic	1 teaspoon
butter	55 g
pumpkin chunks	500 g

vegetable stock	500 ml
coconut cream	400 ml
salt and pepper to taste	

Directions:
1. Peel and dice the onion, after this garlic and mince it (or press – as you wish).
2. Peel the ginger and crush it.
3. Wash and cut the pumpkin. Take off the seeds.
4. Put all the ingredients into the Crock Pot – diced onions, garlic, butter, vegetable stock, pepper and salt at will, pumpkin chunks, crushed ginger.
5. Cover and cook on LOW for 6-7 hours or on HIGH for 5-6 hours.
6. After the time is over, take the cover off, puree the mixture in the blender until smooth consistency.
7. Put on WARM until ready and serve!
8. Garnish with coconut cream.
9. Bon Appetite!

Keto cabbage soup Crock Pot

Never cooked a cabbage soup in the Crock Pot? It is rather easy and tasty dish! You may think: «What is the reason this recipe is included in the cookbook? » This soup is simple to prepare, tasty to eat corresponds to your keto diet, doesn't need great cooking skills, just basic one. Everything you need – to follow the recipe and carry off all the measurements!

Ingredients (8 servings):

Ground beef	2 pounds
Onion	¼ pcs large
Garlic	1 clove
cumin ground	1 teaspoon
cabbage	1 head large
bouillon	4 cubes
Diced tomatoes & green chilies	10 oz can
Water	4 cups

Salt and pepper to taste

Directions:

1. Peel the yellow onion diced it into a bowl. Peel the garlic, press it into the bowl or mince. Chop the cabbage, adding it to the same bowl where the onion is.
2. Brown the ground beef a little over high heat. After some minutes, add the onion, cook in the same skillet until translucent.
3. Put the ground beef in the Crock Pot, add there the browned onion, bouillon.
4. Add to the Crock Pot pressed or minced garlic, chopped cabbage, ground cumin, diced tomatoes, green chilies, water to the Crock Pot.

5. Stir all the ingredients thoroughly, cover the Crock Pot and bring them to boil over the high heat. It takes you about 5 hours.
6. After the time is over (5 hours), reduce it to medium-low, the soup must simmer for 30 minutes on LOW.
7. Add pepper and salt at will.
8. Serve warm.
9. Bon Appetite!

Keto Beef Stroganoff soup Crock Pot

For those who have always loved to cook the beef stroganoff at home or to taste it at the restaurants. There is no other better way to taste the delicious and tender beef in a classic variation. Spice the beef with onion and garlic, add paprika or black pepper at will. Warm, flavorful, savory, spoon after spoon… Mmm, it's delicious! I think this soup idea is a great one!

Ingredients (12 servings):

beef rump steaks	2 large pcs
ghee or lard	¼ cup
garlic	2 cloves
white onion	1 pcs medium

bone broth (it may be also chicken or vegetable stock) 5 cups

paprika	2 teaspoon
Dijon mustard (or homemade)	1 tablespoon
juice of lemon	1 pcs
sour cream (it could be also heavy whipping cream) 1 ½ cup	
freshly parsley	¼ cup
salt	1 teaspoon
ground black pepper	¼ teaspoon

Optionally, a thickener could be used: take 1 tablespoon ground chia seeds or arrowroot powder at will. Mix everything in a ¼ cup warm water or use cream and egg yolk mixture.

Directions:
1. Prepare two beef rump steaks and put them in the freezer in a single layer (for 40 minutes). This procedure makes the steaks to cut them easily into thin strips. After 40 minutes, take a keen knife and slice the steaks into thin strips. Season them with pepper and salt.
2. Peel the white onion, chop it carefully. Peel the garlic and mince.
3. Squeeze the juice of 1 lemon in a cup (it must be about 4 tablespoons).
4. Wash and chop the fresh parsley into a plate.
5. Take a large skillet with a heavy bottom, grease with a half of lard or ghee. Once the skillet is

hot, add the beef slices, but only in a single layer. Fry them over a high heat until brown and take them off to the plate. Do the same with remaining beef slices. Combine them in the plate altogether.

6. Take a bowl with a bone broth, add there paprika, Dijon mustard, salt, and pepper and mix everything. Add the lemon juice, browned beef slices, onion, and garlic. Cover and cook on LOW in the Crock Pot for 3 hours.

7. After the time is over, open the Crock Pot and add sour cream, freshly chopped parsley and ground black pepper. Keep on WARM for 30 minutes.

8. If you use a thickener, add this mixture at the end of the same rule.

9. Eat the dish hot with a slice of keto bread. It could be also cooled in the fridge and stored up to 5 days!

10. Bon Appetite!

Keto Chicken Bacon Chowder

The keto chicken bacon chowder is beyond belief! If you are going to strike your relatives and friends, or your lover with your cooking skills, this is the right choice to prepare. This chowder could be well kept in the refrigerator for 4-5 days. A mix of vegetables and chicken make this combination amazing!

Ingredients (15 servings):

Garlic	4 cloves
shallot	1 pcs medium
leek	1 small
celery	2 ribs
sweet onion	1 pcs medium
butter	4 tablespoons
chicken broth	2 cups
chicken breasts	1 lb
cream cheese	8 oz
heavy cream	1 cup
bacon, cooked crisp and crumbled	1 lb
sea salt	1 teaspoon
black pepper	1 teaspoon
powder of garlic	1 teaspoon
thyme dried	1 teaspoon

Directions:

1. Peel the garlic and mince it carefully. Peel the shallot, chop it finely. Clean the leek, trim and slice. Wash and dice the celery. Peel the sweet onion also, wash and slice it.

2. Divide the chicken broth into two cups. Do the same with butter.
3. Prepare your Crock Pot, add there shallot, garlic, celery, leek, onion, 2 tablespoons of butter, chicken broth (1 cup), season with a little bit pepper and salt to taste.
4. Cap and cook on LOW for 1 hour.
5. While the veggies are cooked, prepare the chicken pieces – wash and cut them thoroughly.
6. Open your Crock Pot and add cut chicken breasts, add also cream cheese, cream, black pepper and salt, garlic powder, dried thyme, chicken broth, bacon strips. Mix plenty all the components. Cap and cook on LOW for 6-7 hours.
7. Serve warm.
8. Bon Appetite!

Keto Crock Pot Cream of Broccoli Soup

This is the soup season! The easy combination of vegetables with cheddar cheese is amazing! The keto cream of broccoli soup is the best way to add healthy vegetables to your daily life during cold and long winter days. Cauliflower and broccoli are full of vitamins, their superpower is incredible of which you might be not aware!

Ingredients (11 servings):

Ghee (or grass-fed butter, coconut oil)   1 tablespoon

broccoli   4 cups

cauliflower   1 cup

garlic   3 cloves

shallot   1 large pcs

chicken broth or stock   4 cups

sea salt   1.5 teaspoon

black pepper   1/2 teaspoon

turmeric   1/4 teaspoon

coconut milk (you must double this if you don't use the cheese)   1/2 cup

cheddar cheese from pasture-raised cows   4 oz

For garnish (if desired): sliced bacon, parsley, fresh cracked black pepper

Directions:
1. Wash and chop the broccoli and cauliflower into florets. Peel the garlic, slice it. Peel, wash and slice a large shallot.
2. Shred the cheddar cheese onto the plate.
3. Put all the ingredients into the Crock Pot – chopped cauliflower and broccoli, garlic and onion. Add the chicken broth, melted butter or

ghee (or coconut oil), mix everything in a Crock Pot. Season with pepper and salt, turmeric.

4. Cover and cook on LOW for about 5-6 hours. The vegetables must be tender and melt in the mouth. You may cook everything on HIGH for 3 hours.
5. When the time is over, add coconut milk, cheddar cheese and blend the soup with a food processor or blender. The soup is hot that's why be very careful!
6. Serve warm, garnish with chopped parsley, bacon slices, cracked black pepper.
7. Bon Appetite!

Keto Crock Pot Chicken Soup

This soup is an amazing combination of chicken luscious pieces, mixed with veggies. The Crock Pot saves your precious time as well as the energy in the kitchen. Basically, one should just add the chicken to your Crock Pot, pile the onion, add your favorite vegetables that will make a delicious mixture of the ingredients. Sweet peppers and jalapenos give the more substance to this chicken soup. I usually serve this soup with avocado, black pepper at will. Usually, I begin to cook this dish in the early morning, and then I have it ready for dinner.

Ingredients (13 servings):
boneless skinless chicken breasts   1 1/2 lbs.

yellow onion	1 medium
bell pepper	1 pcs medium
jalapeno	1 pcs
garlic	2 cloves
diced tomatoes	1 15-oz. can
chicken stock	2 cups
chili powder	1 tablespoon
cumin	1 tablespoon
dried oregano	1 teaspoon
paprika	1/2 teaspoon
fresh coriander	2 tablespoon
avocado, pitted and sliced	1 pcs medium

Salt and freshly ground pepper, to taste

Directions:
1. Prepare the chicken pieces – take off the bones and skin. Wash the breasts and dry with the paper towel.
2. Peel the onion, wash and dice. Wash the sweet pepper, take off the corns, slice it thinly.
3. Wash the jalapeno, dry it with the paper towel, dice into the bowl. Peel the garlic and mince it. Wash the coriander and mince. Wash the avocado, take off the core, slice.

4. Put the chicken pieces into the Crock Pot, add the onion, sweet pepper sliced, chopped jalapeno, minced garlic on the top of the chicken. After this pour the diced tomatoes as well as chicken broth over the top. Season with chili powder, dried cumin, paprika and oregano, pepper, salt.
5. Cap and cook on LOW for 7-8 hours.
6. Once the preparation time is over, open the Crock Pot and using a fork check if the chicken is ready.
7. Serve with fresh chopped coriander and slices of avocado.
8. Bon Appetite!

Pumpkin, Chicken and Spinach Keto Soup

I call this keto soup the Shrek soup because of its yellow-green-mustard color. It is an easy and quick meal that is a fantastic one for those mums who are always busy. The mix of sage, pumpkin, sweetener, a little bit nutmeg allows the dish to be delicious and perfect. This consistency is something between stew and soup.

Ingredients (14 servings):

olive oil   2 tablespoons

chicken breast   1 pound

onion	1 large
garlic	3 large cloves
chicken stock	3-4 cups
pumpkin purée	15 ounce can
sweetener	2 teaspoons
fresh sage leaves	1½ teaspoons
salt	1 teaspoon
freshly ground black pepper	¼ teaspoon
freshly ground nutmeg	⅛ teaspoon
bay leaf	1 pcs
fresh baby spinach leaves	4 cups
fresh lemon juice	1 tablespoon

Dressing: crispy bacon strips

Directions:
1. Prepare the chicken breasts: wash them thoroughly, dry with the paper towel, cut into cubes.
2. Peel the onion and garlic, crush them. Wash the fresh sage leaves, mince them (or use the dried sage leaves). You may roast the minced onion and garlic in 2 tablespoons of olive oil or add these ingredients unroasted to the remained ingredients.

3. Put the chicken pieces into the Crock Pot and stir it with 3 cups of chicken broth. Add there the pumpkin puree, sweetener, pepper, and salt, nutmeg, sage, and bay leaf. Stir everything together.
4. Cover, and cook on LOW for 3 hours.
5. Open the Crock Pot after the time is over, add fresh minced spinach leaves, add ground nutmeg, ground black pepper, salt.
6. Cover the Crock Pot again, turn on WARM and let the leaves wilt. (about 1-2 minutes). After this stir in the fresh lemon juice.
7. Serve warm! Dress with crispy bacon strips.
8. Bon Appetite!

Jalapeno Popper Keto Soup

When the weather is wet and cool I try to eat warm and delicious dishes to let my soul and stomach get warm. This soup is, in general, a one pot meal, keto-friendly and adapted for my great helper – the Crock Pot. My family always enjoys this one, tasting all spicy and hot ingredients. I'm sure enough you'll like it very much. The great thing about this soup, you may add here your favorite species to make it hotter or vice versa.

Ingredients (17 servings):

boneless skinless chicken breasts   1 1/2 lbs

butter   3 tablespoons

garlic minced	2 cloves
onion chopped	½ pcs
green pepper	1/2
jalapenos	2 pcs
bacon crumbled and cooked	1/2 lb
cream cheese	6 oz
chicken broth	3 cups
heavy whipping cream	1/2 cup
paprika	1/4 teaspoon
cumin	1 teaspoon
salt	1 teaspoon
pepper	1/2 teaspoon
Swiss Cheese	3/4 cup
Cheddar Cheese	3/4 cup
xanthan gum	1/2 teaspoon

Directions:
1. Peel the onion and garlic, mince them and put in a bowl.
2. Prepare the chicken breasts – wash them and cut. Shred the Swiss cheese and cheddar.
3. Wash the green pepper, take off the seeds, dry with a paper towel.

4. Wash and dry with a paper towel jalapeno, take off the seeds. Chop carefully.
5. Put the chicken breasts into the Crock Pot, add chicken broth, butter, onion and garlic, chopped jalapenos, green pepper, salt, cumin, paprika, and pepper.
6. Cover and cook on HIGH for 3-4 hours or on LOW on 5-7 hours.
7. After the cooking time is over, take off the chicken, cut into small pieces, and add to the Crock Pot again.
8. Turn the Crock Pot on WARM, open the cover and add cream cheese, heavy whipping cream, cooked bacon (a half of it). Cheese must be melted.
9. At the end of the preparation, sprinkle xanthan gum on the top of your dish, allow it to simmer a little bit on LOW or on WARM for 10 minutes. Let the soup reach the thick consistency.
10. Serve warm with shredded cheese, bacon strips and parsley at will.

Keto Cabbage-Pork Crock Pot

I like to cook soups because this meal is first, a delicious one, secondly, it is essential one, and third – you don't need to wash too many dishes after it! Moreover, cooking the essential meal like cabbage-pork Crock Pot you don't need to prepare each day the new dish – this delicious one will be enough for 2-

3 days. This soup is something fabulous, reach on flavor without carbs. You may also add cauliflower (riced). But it is also great without it.

Ingredients (12 servings):

onion diced	½ pcs medium
garlic minced	2 cloves
pork	1 1/2 lbs
broth (homemade or buy at the store)	3 cups
diced tomatoes	1 14 oz can
tomato sauce	1 8 oz can
Bragg's Aminos	1/4 cup
cabbage chopped	1 small/medium
Worcestershire Sauce	3 teaspoon
Parsley	1/2 teaspoon
Salt	1/2 teaspoon
Pepper	1/2 teaspoon

Directions:
1. Peel garlic and onion and slice them thoroughly.
2. Prepare the pork slices – wash and cut them, drain the water.
3. Cut the cabbage. Wash the parsley and chop.

4. Put the pork slices into the Crock Pot, add sliced onion and garlic, tomato sauce, diced tomatoes from the can, broth, Bragg's Aminos, Worcestershire Sauce, pepper and salt, chopped fresh parsley.
5. Cover and cook on HIGH for 6-7 hours, on LOW for 3-4 hours.
6. The cabbage and the pork must reach the desired tenderness it means the soup is ready.
7. Serve with fresh parsley.
8. Bon Appetite!

Keto Crock Pot Pizza Soup

This keto pizza soup is awesome! I have cooked it several times already! It is something amazing on a plate! I use my favorite sausages, pepperoni, Parmesan and mozzarella cheeses, delicious and hot species. You may also add fresh dill or parsley at the end of cooking process.

Ingredients (12 servings):
crushed tomatoes (can use whole or stewed)
    1 (16 ounces) can

beef broth	2 (16 ounces) cans
olives	2 (16 ounces) cans
green pepper	1 pcs medium
onion	1 small

Italian sausage	1 lb
Pepperoni	1/2 lb
garlic powder	1 teaspoon
dried oregano	2 teaspoons
Italian seasoning	2 teaspoons
mozzarella cheese	1 cup
Parmesan cheese	1/4 cup

Pepper and salt to taste

Directions:
1. Wash and dry the green pepper, take off the corns. Slice the pepperoni thinly. Peel the onion and crush.
2. Cut the sausages.
3. Grate the mozzarella cheese and Parmesan cheese.
4. Put the sausages into the Crock Pot, add crushed tomatoes, beef broth, crushed olives, crushed green pepper and pepperoni, onion, dried oregano, garlic powder, pepper and salt to taste.
5. Cover and cook on LOW for 6-7 hours.
6. Once the time is over, add crushed or shredded Parmesan and mozzarella cheese.
7. Serve warm and enjoy!

Chapter 7: Side Dishes

Mashed Cauliflower with Chives and Parmesan Cheese

Cauliflower is a healthy ingredient and great substitute for potatoes and other vegetables full of carbohydrates. Firstly, this new recipe doesn't appear so delicious, tender and creamy. But if you follow my instructions, you'll get the tender texture of cauliflower with chicken broth (you may also use vegetable one), joined with grated cheese and also chives.
Remember, that potato isn't as healthy as you think.
Just say «hello» to your new friend – cauliflower!

Ingredients (4 servings):

Cauliflower	2 small heads
chicken broth	2 cups
Parmesan cheese	¼ cup
fresh chives	¼ cup
Kosher salt	

ground black pepper at will

Directions:
1. Wash the cauliflower, remove the leaves and core, cut it into small pieces (florets).
2. Grate the Parmesan cheese on a plate. Set aside.
3. Wash and chop the fresh chives.
4. Take a bowl medium-size, combine the cauliflower florets and two cups of chicken broth.
5. Pour it into the Crock Pot, cover and set on LOW for 1 hour, until the cauliflower florets get tender It must not fall apart. Be attentive!
6. Once the time is over, use a long spoon and take off the cauliflower to a blender if you have in a food processor. Puree cauliflower until smooth texture.
7. Transfer mashed cauliflower into a small bowl and stir in the grated Parmesan and fresh chives.
8. Season with salt at will and ground pepper.
9. Serve warm.

Keto Rosemary Garlic Cauliflower

You may ask me, what do we prepare this side dish for? The mashed cauliflower recipe is frequently compared with mashed potatoes. It has a similar texture, consistency and conjoined with similar foods.

But wait, it tastes quite different! Cauliflower isn't the same product as a potato. Both taste amazing, but don't forget about your ketogenic diet! I hope you give this recipe a try.

Ingredients (5 servings):

Cauliflower	1 large
fat cream cheese	3 ounces
unsalted butter	2 tablespoons
minced garlic	1 1/2 teaspoon
fresh rosemary	1 tablespoon

salt and pepper at will

Directions:
1. Wash the cauliflower, remove the leaves and core, cut it into small pieces (florets).
2. Peel the garlic and mince it. You may saute it if you prefer.
3. Wash the rosemary and chop into small pieces.
4. Open the Crock Pot and put the cauliflower florets into, add a little bit water (1/2 cup), cover and put on LOW for 1 hour.
5. Once the time is ready (the cauliflower florets must be tender), remove them from the Crock Pot and let them cool a little.
6. Put the cooked cauliflower in a food processor or a blender, add fat cream cheese, unsalted butter, minced garlic, chopped rosemary and salt if desired. Blend until smooth texture.

7. Serve cool.
8. Bon Appetite!

Squeak and Bubble Crock Pot

This English side dish I cooked firstly because I simply liked the name. This traditional recipe is cooked of cauliflower puree, cabbage, roasted and chopped bacon, scallions and Cheddar cheese. So easy and so perfect!

Ingredients (5 servings) :

cauliflower puree	2 cups
cabbage	1 cup
scallion, green only	1/4 cup
salt & pepper to taste	
cooked bacon	1/4 cup
Cheddar cheese	2 oz

Directions:

Prepare the cauliflower puree:

1. Wash the cauliflower, remove the leaves and core, cut it into small pieces (florets).
2. Open the Crock Pot and put the cauliflower florets into, add a little bit water (1/2 cup), cover and put on LOW for 1 hour.

3. Once the time is ready (the cauliflower florets must be tender), remove them from the Crock Pot and let them cool a little.
4. Put the cooked cauliflower in a food processor and blend until smooth texture.
5. Shred the cabbage and steam it for some minutes until softened.
6. Chop the washed scallions.
7. Join the cabbage with the cauliflower puree and scallions, dress with salt and pepper.
8. Shred the Cheddar cheese and chop the bacon.
9. Put in the Crock Pot, season with shredded cheese and put on LOW for 1 hour.
10. Serve with chopped bacon on top.
11. Bon Appetite!

Cheddar Cauliflower Bacon Bites

Thinking about more recipes for the side dishes? Here you are! A light mix of cauliflower florets, Cheddar cheese, flour and bacon strips! Light, easy, quick and tasty! I think it is the best way to follow your keto diet and prepare in the Crock Pot. And what about you?

Ingredients (8 servings):

cauliflower florets	4 cups
bacon crisps	6 ounces

egg	1 pcs
baking soda	1 teaspoon
salt	1/4 teaspoon
scallions	1/3 cup
coconut flour	1/2 cup
Cheddar cheese	1 cup

Salt at will

Directions:
1. Wash the cauliflower, remove the leaves and core, cut it into large pieces (florets).
2. Open the Crock Pot and put the cauliflower florets into, add a little bit water (1/2 cup), cover and put on LOW for 1 hour.
3. Once the time is ready (the cauliflower florets must be tender), remove them from the Crock Pot and let them cool a little.
4. Put the cooked cauliflower in a food processor and blend until smooth texture.
5. Wash and chop the scallions. Shred the Cheddar cheese and set aside.
6. Take a large bowl, mix the cauliflower with salt, add cracked egg, chopped scallions, coconut flour, baking soda. Mix everything well.
7. Spray the bottom and sides of the Crock Pot with cooking spray and put the mixture into it.
8. Cover the Crock Pot and put on HIGH for 1 hour.

9. Once the time is over, put the bacon crisps on the top and spread the shredded Cheddar cheese. Cover and put on WARM for one additional hour.
10. Serve warm and enjoy immediately!
11. Bon Appetite!

Creamy Greek Zucchini Crock Pot

This creamy Greek zucchini side dish is flavor and tender. This recipe is a set of health, spring, color, and taste. I advise you to use only the organic eggs, fresh herbs that you may buy at the farmers' shops and fresh feta cheese. You may also change Feta with the other cheese you prefer more.

Ingredients (9 servings):

zucchini	2 lbs (about 7 large)
organic eggs	2 large
fresh herbs	1 cup
almond meal (or keto breadcrumbs)	1 cup
feta cheese	1 cup
ground cumin	1 teaspoon
fine grain sea salt	1 teaspoon

Ground black pepper at will

olive oil   3 tablespoons

Directions:
1. Wash zucchini, take off the ends.
2. Put them in a blender and grate.
3. Put the grated zucchini in a medium bowl and season with salt. Leave them to drain for 30 minutes.
4. Take handfuls of the grated zucchini, squeeze all of the moisture. Set aside.
5. Take a medium bowl, beat eggs, add zucchini, cumin, herbs, meal. Mix everything. Add salt, feta, and pepper. Stir well.
6. Place the ready mixture in the refrigerator for 30 minutes.
7. Open the Crock Pot, spread the cooking spray or olive oil over the bottom and sides.
8. Put the mixture into the Crock Pot and set on HIGH for 1 hour.
9. Remove the side dish once the time is over.
10. Serve!

Crock Pot Keto Cheesy Zucchini

Speaking about keto side dishes, I must say, I like light vegetable variations in creamy-cheesy combinations. This recipe recommended as a side dish, prepared in the Crock Pot is a really creative combination of cheese (you may also choose Swiss or parmesan cheese) milk, butter and zucchini noodles. Let's try to cook!

Ingredients (6 servings):

Zucchini	1 pcs
Water	1/2 cup
Salt	1 teaspoon
Butter	1 tablespoon
Milk	2 tablespoon
Cheddar cheese	2/3 - 1 cup

black pepper at will

Directions:
1. Wash the zucchini, dry with a paper towel. Cut the ends of it and with a help of spiralizer make „noodles ".
2. Take a saucepan medium-sized, put the noodles into a saucepan, add water, season with salt and let them boil. Noodles must get soft.
3. Shred the Cheddar cheese.
4. Remove the noodles from the Crock Pot, butter, milk, pepper and shredded cheese.
5. Cover and cook on LOW for 30 minutes.
6. Serve warm, add if desired black pepper!
7. Bon Appetite!

Chapter 8: Vegetarian and Vegan

Crock Pot Vegetable Soup

This recipe of vegetable soup is excellent for calming the nervous system. You may also add the other herbs according to your own tastes or tastes of your family. Blend the mixture until smooth once the cooking time is over.

Ingredients (11 servings):

Cauliflower	1 head
Watercress	½ cup
olive oil	2 tablespoons
sweet onion	1 medium
leek	1pcs
celery 1 stalk	
water (or vegetable stock)	6 cups
bay leaf	1 pcs

thyme   1 branch

sea salt   2 pinches

dill   1/4 cup

black pepper at will

Directions:
1. Peel and chop the onion. Set aside.
2. Chop the leek, celery, dill.
3. Chop finely the cauliflower.
4. Take a medium-sized skillet, heat the olive oil over medium heat.
5. Add onion, leeks, celery into the skillet and cauliflower florets. Cook about 5 minutes, the onions must be translucent.
6. Add water thyme, and salt at will, bay leaf to the Crock Pot, pour the ready-made veggies from the skillet.
7. Cover the Crock Pot and set on HIGH for 3 hours.
8. Using a blender blend the soup until smooth mix.
9. Add black pepper or cilantro and serve.
10. Dress with watercress.
11. Bon Appetite!

Crock Pot Broccoli Tofu Soup

This easy Crock Pot recipe is great if you need a healthy meal but you don't have time to prepare this meal. It is quick, healthy, full of minerals and vitamins, keto-friendly and tasty! Add Tofu cheese for garnish or fresh basil leaves!

Ingredients (9 servings):

broccoli florets	5 cups (about 16 ounces)
yellow onion	1 medium
garlic	3 cloves
dried oregano	1 teaspoon
freshly grated nutmeg	1/4 teaspoon
vegetable broth	2 1/2 cups
kosher salt	1/2 teaspoon
black pepper	1/4 teaspoon
Tofu cheese low-carb	1 (8-ounce) block

Directions:
1. Peel the onion and slice finely.
2. Peel the garlic and mince.
3. Chop the broccoli florets.
4. Open the Crock Pot and put the broccoli, onion, and garlic in the bottom of the Crock Pot. Add oregano, nutmeg, and vegetable broth.
5. Add Tofu. Cover the Crock Pot and set on HIGH for 2 hours.
6. Once the cooking time is over, use the blender and puree the soup, it must be of smooth consistency.

7. Serve warm. Season with fresh parsley or grated Tofu.
8. Bon Appetite!

Easy Vegetarian Roasted Chestnut Soup

I know that not everybody likes chestnuts, but if you still like, you will definitely cook this soup recipe! This vegan chestnut soup is delicious and light. I advise you to check the soymilk when you will buy it at the store as some kinds of them contain sugar.

Ingredients (9 servings):

olive oil	3 tbsp. vegan
celery	1 rib
onion	1 pcs
strong vegetable broth	6 cups
fresh parsley	1/4 cup
ground cloves	1/4 tsp.
bay leaves	2 pcs
chestnuts (roasted and peeled)	12 oz.
unsweetened soymilk	1/4 cup

Salt and pepper at will

Directions:

1. Mince celery. Peel the onion and mince.
2. Wash the parsley and chop.
3. Peel and the cloves and mince finely.
4. Peel and roast the chestnuts.
5. Take a large saucepan, saute minced garlic, celery, onion with oil until softened, about 7 minutes.
6. Open the Crock Pot, add vegetable broth. Add chopped fresh parsley, cloves, bay leaves and the chestnuts. Put the mixture in the skillet. Add soymilk.
7. Toss everything well. Put the Crock Pot on HIGH for 3 hours.
8. Once the cooking time is over, take off the bay leaves, using a blender make a puree.
9. Dress with salt and pepper before serving.
10. Bon Appetite!

Crock Pot Easy Keto Soup

You know, something happens to fresh vegetables usually when they are cooked slowly for a long time in the Crock Pot. Your kitchen is full of aromas and the veggie soup is super tender and light!

Ingredients (5 servings):

Leeks	8 oz (225 g)
spinach	8 oz

onion   1 pcs small

vegetable stock   2½ pints

bay leaves   2 pcs

salt and black pepper at will

fresh chives for garnish

Directions:
1. Trim and wash the leeks, cut into 2-inch pieces.
2. Peel chop finely the onions.
3. Wash and cut the spinach.
4. Open the Crock Pot and put the leeks, onion, bay leaves, dressed with pepper and salt. Add vegetable stock.
5. Cover the lid and put on LOW for 3 hours.
6. When the time is almost finished, open the lid and put spinach.
7. Serve warm fresh chives, dress with pepper and salt.
8. Bon Appetite!

Italian Vegetable Keto Bake

An Italian vegetable dish prepared in the Crock Pot, full with sunny courgettes, tomatoes, herbs, and aubergine is irresistible! You may cook this keto dish for parties as an addition to the main dish or eat it without anything.

Ingredients (7 servings):

garlic	3 cloves
tomato	1 can
bunch oregano	
pinch chili flakes	
baby aubergines	11oz
Courgettes	2 pcs
roasted red peppers	½ large jar
beef tomatoes	3 pcs
bunch basil if desired	
green salad at will	

Directions:
1. Peel the garlic and mince.
2. Chop tomatoes from the can
3. Wash the courgettes and slice, chop baby aubergines. Slice beef tomatoes.
4. Open the Crock Pot, put the garlic, chopped tomatoes, oregano leaves, chili and some seasoning, add olive oil if necessary.
5. Add chopped aubergines, tomatoes, courgettes, red peppers, basil and remaining oregano. Repeat vegetable layer, herb, and tomatoes. Push down well to compress, set on HIGH for 5 hours.

6. Serve with the basil leaves and the green
    salad.
7. Bon Appetite!

Crock Pot Vegetarian Stew Keto Recipe

One of my favorite flavor vegetarian stews is this one. If you want to get
the creamy texture of it, use the blender or the food processor you have at home and blend the stew at the end of the cooking.

Ingredients (11 servings):

Onion   1 medium pcs

Celery   1 stalk

Kale   4 cup

garlic   4 clove

Italian Seasoning   1 teaspoon

diced tomatoes   1 can

pumpkin   2 cups canned

chicken broth 4 cup

chicken breast   2 breast

sea salt   1/8 teaspoon

black pepper, ground 1/8 teaspoon

Directions:
1. Peel the onions, chop finely.
2. Chop the leek. Chop the kale.
3. Peel the garlic and mince.
4. Open the Crock Pot and put everything into the Crock Pot, cover the lid and set on LOW for 7 hours.
5. Once the time is over, serve the dish tor and season additionally with black pepper.
6. Bon Appetite!

Chapter 9: Dessert Recipes

White Chocolate Green Tea Mug Keto Cake

Green tea mug keto cake is one of my lovely and unusual cakes ever. Firstly, I tried it in the restaurant, its colored has surprised me at once! But what an amazing taste it has! I cooked it at home and found it was nothing difficult to prepare. The only necessary ingredient you have to put there is matcha powder. This ingredient makes the dessert flavorful, decadent, rich and funny!

Ingredients (11 servings):

powdered erythritol	1.5 tablespoon
liquid stevia	5-10 drops
egg	1 large
coconut oil (or melted butter)	1 tablespoon
vanilla extract	1/2 teaspoon
almond flour	1/4 cup

matcha powder	1/2 teaspoon
baking powder	1 teaspoon
xanthan gum	1/8 teaspoon
sea salt	1 pinch

frozen sugar-free white chocolate chips 2 tablespoon

Directions:
1. Freeze the sugar-free white chocolate chips beforehand to ensure they stay as chips while baking.
2. Open the Crock Pot and spread the cooking spray over the sides and the bottom.
3. Take a large bowl, whisk the erythritol and stevia into the egg.
4. Add the coconut oil (or if you use the butter - melted butter) and vanilla extract and whisk everything well to combine.
5. In another medium-sized bowl combine together almond flour, matcha powder, baking powder and xanthan gum.
6. Add this mix to the other wet ingredients. Add also a pinch salt, combine everything very well.
7. Fold in the white chocolate chips.
8. Pour in the Crock Pot, cover and set on LOW for 2 hours.
9. Once the baking time is over, let the cake cool and enjoy!
10. Bon Appetite!

Keto Peanut Butter Cake

Peanut butter cake has a special place among my keto desserts prepared in the Crock Pot. There are only three ingredients needed for the cake. They are the sweetener, peanut butter, and a fresh egg. It is simple enough, even kids can prepare this delicious cake.

Ingredients (3 servings):

peanut butter   1 cup

granular erythritol   1/2 cup

egg   1 large

Directions:

1. Open the Crock Pot and spread the cooking spray over the sides and the bottom.
2. Blend a half of an amount of granular erythritol into a food processor and blend for some seconds. You should get a finely powdered sweetener.
3. In a medium-sized bowl combine peanut butter with powdered erythritol and the fresh egg, mix everything well.
4. Roll the cake into a medium-sized ball and place on a bottom of the Crock Pot.
5. Cover the Crock Pot and set on LOW for 3 hours. Check the readiness from time to time, the cake edges must turn a darker brown.
6. Once the baking time is over, take off the cake and let it cool.

7. Enjoy with a glass of milk!

Black and White Keto Cake

An amazing keto cake that consists of chocolate and… chocolate! White and black! Always more chocolate for chocolate fans! Yes, I'm sure, you will not forget this texture! Don't forget to use sugar-free and keto-friendly ingredients in this recipe! It is a perfect alternative to sweets and chocolate!

Ingredients (16 servings):
For Cake

Almond flour	2 cups
coconut flour	2 tablespoon
sweetener	1 cup
baking soda	1.5 teaspoon
salt	1/2 teaspoon
butter	1 cup
cocoa powder	1/2 cup
water	1 cup
eggs	3 large
vanilla extract	2 teaspoon
sour cream	1/2 cup

White Chocolate Glaze:

Cocoa Butter Wafers   2 oz.

powdered erythritol   3 tablespoon

vanilla extract   1 teaspoon

heavy cream   2 tablespoon

Topping

Cocoa Nibs   20 grams

Directions:
1. Open the Crock Pot and spread the cooking spray over the sides and the bottom.
2. In a medium-sized bowl whisk together almond flour with coconut flour, sweetener baking soda, and salt. Set aside.
3. Take a small pot, heat together butter, cocoa powder, water on a high heat. Whisk everything until combined and take it off from the heat.
4. Pour a half of chocolate mixture into dry ingredients (first bowl) and stir to combine. Once the mixture is thick and difficult to stir, pour the other half. Combine once more.
5. Add in 1 egg, after this add sour cream and vanilla extract, stir everything well.
6. Pour the batter into the Crock Pot and set on LOW for 5 hours, until the wooden toothpick comes out clean.
7. While the cake is baking, it is time to prepare white chocolate glaze.

8. In a little saucepan melt cocoa butter wafers.
9. Add powdered erythritol and mix to combine.
10. Add heavy cream and put the mixture in the fridge, stirring every 6-7 minutes.
11. Once the chocolate has chilled to the thick consistency, pulse it for some seconds in a blender until smooth.
12. Once the cake is ready, let it cool for about 10 minutes, then put it on a plate and let it cool completely.
13. After this glaze the cake. Let the glaze drape over the top of the cake.
14. Dress with the nibs.
15. Enjoy!

Keto pumpkin cake Crock Pot

Keto pumpkin cake prepared in the Crock Pot is great for everyday desserts. It is delicious creamy pumpkin base with a coffee cake crumble flavor topping. I'm sure, it will magically disappear from the kitchen once it is ready!

Ingredients (16 servings):

coconut flour	1/3 cup
pumpkin pie spice	2 teaspoon
cinnamon	1 teaspoon
salt	1/8 teaspoon

eggs	2 pcs
organic pumpkin puree	1/3 cup
sweetener	1/3 cup
coconut milk	1/4 cup
coconut oil	2 tablespoon
vanilla extract	1 teaspoon
baking soda	½ teaspoon

Crumble Topping:

pecan meal	1/2 cup
coconut flakes	3 tablespoon
coconut sugar	2 tablespoon
cinnamon	1 teaspoon
coconut oil	3 tablespoon

Directions:

1. Open the Crock Pot and spread the cooking spray over the sides and the bottom.
2. Take a medium-sized mixing bowl and combine coconut flour, pumpkin pie spice, cinnamon, and sea salt. Mix everything thoroughly. Set aside.
3. Take another large mixing bowl and combine eggs, coconut milk, pumpkin puree, melted coconut oil or butter,

sweetener, and vanilla extract. Mix together until combined.

4.   Add baking soda to the egg mixture. Mix together thoroughly.

5.   Add coconut flour mix to the egg mix and stir until combined.

6.   Pour into the Crock Pot and set aside.

7.   In a little bowl combine pecan meal, coconut flakes, coconut sugar, oil, and cinnamon, use a fork to mix until paste forms.

8.   Take the crumble topping all over the top of the pumpkin batter in the Crock Pot.

9.   Cover the Crock Pot and set on LOW for 4 hours until top is browned, and a toothpick comes out clean.

10.   Cool the cake completely, then refrigerate for one hour or longer.

11.   Bon Appetite!

Keto Pumpkin Chocolate Chip

This dessert recipe is something special because of the mix sweet coconut flour, chocolate chips with cardamom, ginger powder and ground cloves. But be sure, it rather tasty, flavor and simple.

Ingredients (13 servings):

almond butter unsweetened   1/2 cup

pumpkin puree unsweetened   1/4 cup

erythritol granulated	1/4 cup
ginger powder	1/4 teaspoon
nutmeg	1/4 teaspoon
cardamon powder	1/4 teaspoon
ground cloves	1/4 teaspoon
cinnamon	1 teaspoon
stevia powder	1/4 teaspoon
baking soda	1/2 teaspoon
coconut flour	1 tablespoon
chocolate chips	2 tablespoon
egg	1pcs

Directions:

1. Open the Crock Pot and spread the cooking spray over the sides and the bottom.
2. Mix in a large bowl pumpkin puree, almond butter, sweetener, ginger powder, nutmeg, cardamom powder, freshly cracked egg, ground cloves, cinnamon, stevia powder, baking soda, coconut flour. Stir everything well.
3. Add chocolate chips.
4. Put the mixture into the Crock Pot, cover and set on HIGH for 2 hours.
5. Take out and let it cool.

6.   Bon Appetite!

Keto Crock Pot Cheesecake

When I tried to cook this recipe for the first time I couldn't believe the cheesecake could be so easy!!!! It is amazing, flavor and tender cake! I think I don't need to tell you more about the cheesecake. You may serve it with low carb fruit sauce, berries. The best way – to let it cool in the refrigerator for a night, but I can't stand it!

Ingredients (4 servings):

cream cheese	3 8 oz. packages
eggs	3 pcs
Splenda	1 cup
Vanilla	½ tablespoon

Directions:
1. Let the cheese (cream cheese) get the room temperature. Place it in a medium-sized bowl, add Splenda.
2. Using a blender mix everything well, until cheese and Splenda are blended thoroughly.
3. Add the cracked eggs, one after one blending all the time the mixture.
4. Spray the bottom and the sides of the Crock Pot with cooking spray, pour the egg-cheese mixture into the Crock Pot.

5. Cover and put the dish on HIGH for 2 hours.
6. Look after an hour from time to time. Check the readiness of the cheesecake – the knife must go out from the cake clean.
7. Let it cool.
8. Bon Appetite!

Keto Crock Pot Pumpkin Custard

This pumpkin custard is one of my favorite because it is baked in the Crock Pot. It is very flavorful and creamy. I just mix all the ingredients in a large bowl, blend well and after this pour to the Crock Pot. I usually use Stevia in my recipes (blended variation) or you may use another sweetener if you want. Instead of the vanilla extract, you may use the maple syrup if you like.

Ingredients (8 servings):

Eggs	4 large
granulated stevia	1/2 cup
pumpkin puree (canned)	1 cup
vanilla extract	1 teaspoon
superfine almond flour	1/2 cup
pumpkin pie spice	1 teaspoon
sea salt	1/8 teaspoon

butter, ghee	4 tablespoons

Directions:

1. Blend the granulated Stevia. Set aside.
2. Break the eggs into a bowl, compound them until smooth consistency (the mix must thicken slightly). Add a little bit the vanilla extract, put the pumpkin puree. Combine everything well once more.
3. Add slowly pie spice, salt, flour and stir thoroughly. Go on the blend.
4. Melt butter or ghee, pour slowly into the blended mixture. Stir everything well.
5. Spray the cooking spray over the bottom of the Crock Pot, pour the compound into the Crock Pot.
6. Put the paper towel over the top of the Crock Pot, a cap must be covered. So, it means the towel is arranged between the cap and the top. It must absorb the condensed damp.
7. Put the Crock Pot on LOW for ca. 3 hours. Check from time to time. When the dish is ready, the sides must put off from the Crock Pot.
8. Take off the custard from the Crock Pot, serve with Stevia whipped cream and nutmeg at will.
9. Bon Appetite!

Lemon Crock Pot Cake

This amazing lemon keto cake was prepared during 3 hours without any strong efforts. I must say, this keto cake tasted better the next day as it was kept all the night in the refrigerator. I think the cakes made of coconut or almond flour taste better when you keep them at least some hours in the refrigerator.

Ingredients:

Baking a cake:

almond flour	1 1/2 cup
coconut flour	1/2 cup
Puree all-purpose (or Swerve)	3 teaspoons
baking powder	2 teaspoons
xanthan gum optional	1/2 teaspoon
butter melted	1/2 cup
whipping cream	1/2 cup
Juice of lemon	2 tablespoons
Zest from two lemons	
Eggs	2 pcs

Cooking a topping:

Puree all-purpose (or Swerve)	3 teaspoons
baking powder	2 teaspoons

boiling water	1/2 cup
butter melted	2 tablespoons
lemon juice	2 tablespoons

Directions:

Baking a cake:

1. Take a medium-sized bowl, conjoin the coconut flour, sweetener, almond flour, baking powder, xanthan gum. Stir well everything
2. In another bowl whisk the butter, squeeze the lemon juice, xanthan gum, whipping cream, zest, crack the egg in a bowl.
3. Combine both mixtures dry and wet one.
4. Spray the cooking spray over the Crock Pot, pour the mixture into the Crock Pot. Cover and put on HIGH for 3 hours until the inserted in the center knife comes out clean.
5. While the cake is cooking, prepare the topping – conjoin the baking powder, water, melted butter and lemon juice.
6. Take off the cake once it is ready for a large plate. Pour the topping over it.
7. Add whipped cream or fresh fruits by serving, if desired.
8. Bon Appetite!

Keto Chocolate Cake Crock Pot

This should be definitely the best low carb cake recipe one has ever tried to cook and to eat! It is reach and flavor! I guess, it is no need to describe the chocolate cake prepared in the Crock Pot. It is delicious. Just cook it following the directions below.

Ingredients (10 servings):

almond flour	1 cup and additionally 2 tablespoon
sweetener	1/2 cup
cocoa powder	1/2 cup
whey protein powder	3 tablespoon
baking powder	1 1/2 teaspoon
salt	1/4 teaspoon
eggs	3 large pcs
butter melted	6 tablespoon
unsweetened almond milk	2/3 cup
vanilla extract	3/4 teaspoon

Directions:

1. Spray the bottom and all the sides of the Crock Pot with cooking spray.
2. Take a bowl, mix well the almond flour, cocoa powder, sweetener, protein powder, baking powder, salt. Stir everything well.

3. Add butter (melted), cracked eggs, milk, vanilla.
    Combine everything.
4. Pour the ready-made mixture into the Crock
    Pot, cover and put on LOW for ca. 2 hours. It
    must look like a pudding.
5. Take off from the Crock Pot and let it cool.
6. Serve warm with whipping cream.
7. Bon Appetite!

Crock Pot Raspberry-Vanilla Pudding Cake

If you have a small container of fresh raspberries, don't hesitate to cook this amazing cake! It is a flavor, appetizing, tender pudding cake. The mixture is rather simple, it contains egg-free texture with an addition of boiling hot water at the end of cooking process. This dessert is amazing, keto-friendly, simple. Top this cake with vanilla, fresh raspberries and whipping cream.

Ingredients (10 servings):

Sweetener	2 cups
almond flour	2 cups
baking powder	4 teaspoon
salt	1 teaspoon
milk	1 cup

butter	4 tablespoon
vanilla	1 teaspoon
fresh raspberries	2 (6 oz) container
vanilla pudding mix	1 tablespoon
boiling water	1 3/4 cup

some fresh raspberries for dressing

Vanilla or whipped cream

Directions:
1. Take a medium bowl, combine flour, sweetener, baking powder, vanilla, salt, milk. Whisk everything. Melt the butter and add to the mixture.
2. Open the container with raspberries and pour them into the mixture.
3. Spread the cooking spray over the sides and bottom of the Crock Pot.
4. Put the mixture into the Crock Pot and spread it on the bottom.
5. Sprinkle the pudding mix over the top of the mixture but don't stir it.
6. Take a little bowl, let the water boil.
7. Pour the water carefully over the top of the pudding mix and the mixture.
8. Cover and put on HIGH for 2 hours.
9. The ready-made pudding will be on the bottom of the cake.

10. Serve with whipping cream or vanilla and fresh raspberries.
11. Bon Appetite!

Conclusion

Trying something new, for example, new diet, we usually wonder – if the chosen method suitable for me? How can I avoid eating forbidden products? What must I cook today? Is it boring? How many times should I go shopping? It is a total misconception, I think if a person thinks the ketogenic diet is just eating boring food without some variety of recipes and tasty combinations. The recipes of this cookbook contain a huge number of recipes from single portions to full meals that could feed the whole your family and friends, reasoning how easy and tasty could be the keto diet. But what about if you are always in a hurry, busy, have a big family? Maybe you have no mood to cook at all? Is the cooking process boring for you? You don't like washing pile of dishes all the time, don't you? I have gathered all the keto-friendly recipes that you may cook in the Crock Pot! It solves all your problems. No need to spend a lot of time on the stove, no need to search on the Internet for hours trying to follow the keto-rules and keeping in the mind necessary information all the time. I have done all these jobs for you! I think the ketogenic diet is the easiest and simplest way one could choose to burn fat in the body for energy. This cookbook will definitely help you to say «Goodbye» to preferred bread, potatoes, rice and pasta, and to say warm greetings to oils and cheese. The ketogenic diet really works if you follow the rules posted on the food list (forbidden and allowed products) and the genius Crock Pot helps you in the achievement of the aim. Think about your health – Could you do something useful for it right now? Consuming of heart-healthy fats decrease the possible risk of heart diseases, the limitation of sweets and sugar lowers the risk of diabetes type 2. Of course, eating keto-friendly food doesn't mean to consume ice cream or any kind of fat all the time. There is a huge variety of products low in carbohydrates and full of fat that is advised you at the recipes of this keto Crock Pot cookbook.

Do check out my other books that helps you eat healthier, burn fat & to live an active lifestyle!

Keto Diet Crock Pot Cookbook by Oliver Cooper

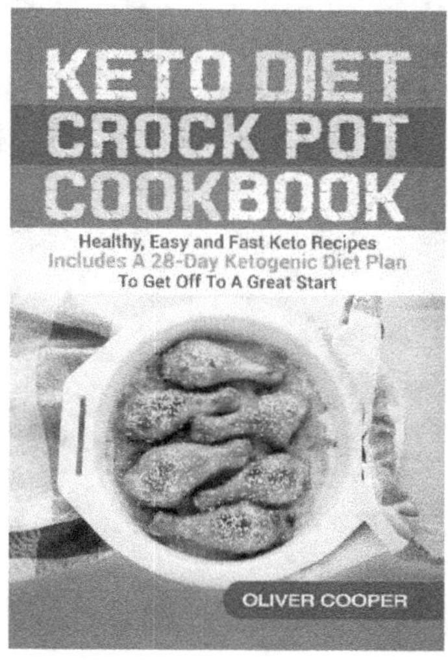

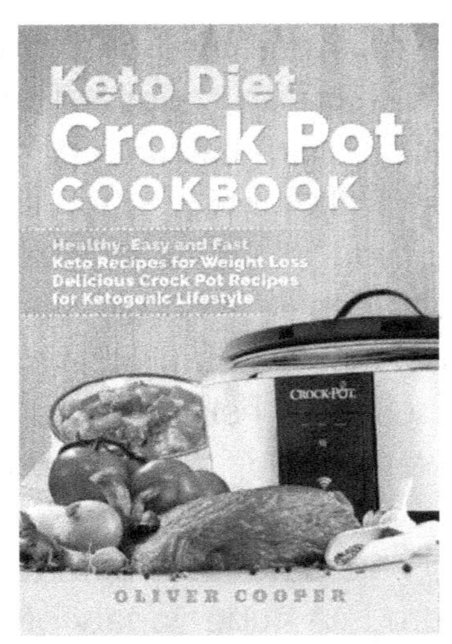

Keto Diet
Crock Pot
COOKBOOK
Healthy, Easy and Fast
Keto Recipes for Weight Loss
Delicious Crock Pot Recipes
for Ketogenic Lifestyle
CROCK-POT
OLIVER COOPER

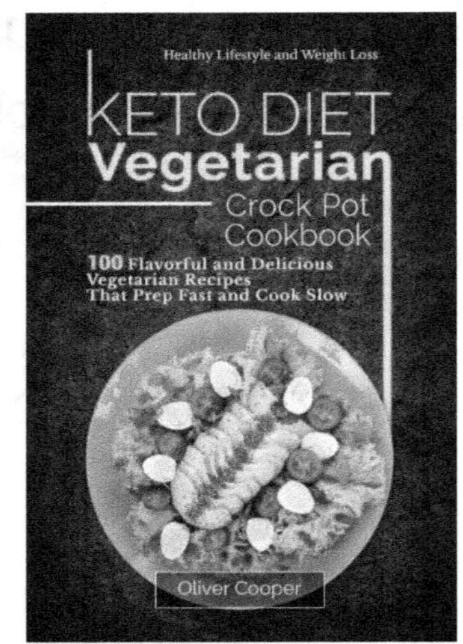

Healthy Lifestyle and Weight Loss
KETO DIET
Vegetarian
Crock Pot
Cookbook
100 Flavorful and Delicious
Vegetarian Recipes
That Prep Fast and Cook Slow
Oliver Cooper

Author's Afterthoughts

Thanks ever so much to each of my cherished readers for investing the time read this book!

I know you could have picked from many other books but you chose this one. So big thanks for downloading this book and reading all way to the end.

If you enjoyed this book or received value from it, I'd like to ask you for a favor. Please take a few minutes to post an honest and heartfelt review on Amazon.com Your support does make a difference and to benefit other people.

תודה

Dankie Gracias

Спасибо شكراً Merci Takk

Köszönjük Terima kasih

Grazie Dziękujemy Děkojame

Ďakujeme Vielen Dank Paldies

Kiitos Täname teid 谢谢

Thank You Tak

感謝您 Obrigado Teşekkür Ederiz 감사합니다

Σας ευχαριστούμε ขอบคุณ

Bedankt Děkujeme vám

ありがとうございます

Tack